# Thin For Good

Also by Fred Pescatore, M.D.

*Feed Your Kids Well*

# Thin For Good

*The One Low-Carb Diet That*
*Will Finally Work for You*

Fred Pescatore, M.D.

JOHN WILEY & SONS, INC.

New York • Chichester • Weinheim • Brisbane • Singapore • Toronto

Published by John Wiley & Sons, Inc.
Published simultaneously in Canada

Design and production by Navta Associates, Inc.

The information contained in this book is not intended to serve as a replacement for professional medical advice. Any use of the information in this book is at the reader's dis-cretion. The author and the publisher specifically disclaim any and all liability arising directly or indirectly from the use or application of any information contained in this book. A health care professional should be consulted regarding your specific situation.

*Library of Congress Cataloging-in-Publication Data*

Pescatore, Fred
    Thin for good : the one low-carb diet that will finally work for you /
Fred Pescatore.
        p.   cm.
    Includes index.
    ISBN 0-471-36267-0 (cloth : acid-free paper)
    1. Low-carbohydrate diet.   2. Reducing diets.   3. Women—Health and hygiene.   4. Men—Health and hygiene.   I. Title.

RM237.73 .P47   2000
613.2'5—dc21                                                    99-054631

Printed in the United States of America
10  9  8  7  6  5  4  3  2  1

*This book is dedicated to SHF, whose constant inspiration makes it all possible.*

# Author's Note

The information in this book reflects the author's experience and is not intended to replace the advice of your own personal physician. It is not the intent of the author to diagnose or prescribe treatment. The intent is only to help you lose weight and perhaps gain health, in conjunction with your own personal physician. Only your personal physician can determine if this nutritional lifestyle program is suitable for you, depending on your personal medical history. In addition to regular checkups and supervision, any questions or symptoms that may arise should be addressed to your personal physician.

This book is not meant to serve as a replacement for your personal physician. Rather, it should be used as an adjunct or an alternative to what you've been hearing for many years about what to eat.

In the event you use this information without your doctor's approval, you are prescribing for yourself, and the publisher and the author assume no responsibility.

# Contents

## Part IV  The Mind-Body Medicines and the Suggested Thin For Good Meal Plans

## Part V  Your Thin For Good Supplements

## Part VI  Enhancing Thin For Good

## Part VII  Thin For Good Recipes

# Acknowledgments

There are so many people without whom this book would not have been possible. I would like to especially mention the following:

EM for always believing in the project

HE for her contributions to the recipe section. Boy, are they good!

PM, EI, and HC for being themselves

DC for too many things to mention

TM for always being able to get that just right, extra sentence out of me

CS for his dedication, hard work, and patience

And, of course, to my many patients who are a constant source of inspiration and enjoyment.

I couldn't have done this without you. Thanks.

# Introduction

*Thin For Good* provides the missing link to thinness by giving you:

1. a good, healthy low-carbohydrate diet program, and
2. the power to use your mind to control your body.

The way most North Americans are being encouraged to eat today is wrong. There is no scientific evidence to support the claim that by eating a high-carbohydrate, low-fat diet, you will get healthier and thinner. Instead, there is ample evidence to support the fact that a diet too low in fat may eventually lead to adverse health consequences, especially an increase in heart disease—amazingly, the main problem a diet low in fat was supposed to solve.

This "low-fat myth," as I like to call it, has resulted in people believing that they can eat as many carbohydrates as they wish, as long as they don't contain fat. How many times have you sat down and finished an entire box of cookies or an entire pound of pasta and rationalized it by telling yourself that, after all, the food was fat-free? Fat-free maybe, but what about all the sugar you've just ingested? Yes, there is sugar in those fat-free foods. And yet you still expected to lose weight.

Besides, don't you find eating fat-free a little boring? I know I do.

When I decided to write this book, I wanted to keep the good principles of low-carbohydrate eating, leave the bad ones behind, and at the same time change the way people look at food.

*Thin For Good* teaches you to choose *all* the delicious and nutritious foods you may eat—and which foods you should avoid—while still losing weight. *Thin For Good* eliminates a treacherous roadblock on the way to thinness: boredom, by not only being much more varied than most other low-carbohydrate diets but by giving you a mind plan that will leave the boredom behind.

During my years as the Associate Medical Director of the Atkins Center, I realized that the paradigm needed to change. I do not want people relegated to counting carbohydrates their entire lives—a new obsession that for some people has replaced the old obsessions about counting calories or fat grams. The problems with the old low-carb diets were especially evident with women, who found that eating all that meat wasn't enabling them to lose the weight they wanted.

*Thin For Good* offers a new low-carbohydrate way of eating, though not as restrictive as the Atkins diet. I believe it is possible to lose weight without having to be so strict about the carbohydrate content. You won't have to completely ignore carbohydrates that have nutritional value. Just as all fats are not bad, neither are all carbohydrates. I'll show you the differences.

As for fats, you will not be eating an unlimited amount of that food group, either. Fried foods and saturated fats must be limited when trying to devise an eating plan for life. Eating all the bacon and chicken skin you want is not healthy. The Atkins diet rarely took those things into account.

Think about it. How many diets have you been on in your lifetime? If you are an average North American, the number is at least ten. As you read this, one out of three Americans is currently dieting. Some of the diets we go on are pretty loony. And frankly, many of them work—at least in the short term.

In *Thin For Good*, I will also show you how the most important component of being a successful dieter was missing from all the other programs you have ever been on. Simply put, you must have the proper mind-body connection if you are ever going to be successful at dieting. No other diet has given you this information, and that's why you haven't been able to stay thin—*up until now.*

I have developed a concept called "Mind Over Calories." Mind Over Calories will help you understand the rage and frustration you feel every time you follow a diet perfectly and still fail to lose weight. Food plays an extremely powerful role in the psyche. If you doubt this, I encourage you to take a moment to consider your food cravings and how emotional they may make you get from time to time.

*Thin For Good* opens the power of your mind to aid your weight loss, something you will not find in other low-carbohydrate eating plans such as *Protein Power, Sugar Busters,* or *The Zone.* None of those diets focuses on balancing the mind with the body. If you don't include your mind in the dieting process, you are ultimately doomed to failure. *Thin For Good* provides the solution to many of dieting's psychological roadblocks—you won't find it in those other bestsellers.

This book will help you learn how to overcome the overweight mindset, or at least how to have better coping strategies. Ultimately, it will teach you a new way of life. Your mind holds the key to your success. This is what will make this diet work where others have failed.

For each day of *Thin For Good*'s initiation phase, I will give you an inspirational tip to teach you how to overcome your overweight mindset. I'll give you an easy one now: Don't call this a diet; call it a nutritional lifestyle program.

For most of us, the word "diet" makes us think of *deprivation*. As someone who spent most of his childhood and young adulthood as an overweight person, I can tell you that I uttered the phrase, "I can't wait for this diet to be over!" so many times that it practically became my motto. As soon as this diet is over, I can go back to eating the way I like, right? Wrong! You can never be a truly thin person until you stop thinking of a diet as something that has a beginning and an end. Simply put, "diet" must become what you eat.

*Thin For Good* will provide you with the solution you'll need to master in order to never have to "diet" again. You will see that your mind plays an enormous role in this transformation.

Besides the power of the mind-body connection, there is something else I've learned in my years of practicing nutritional medicine: Women and men eat differently. No other diet book has addressed this cornerstone topic. *Thin For Good* provides you with another first, namely, one diet for women and another for men. The two diets are similar in that they draw on the same premise of low-carbohydrate eating, but they take into account the fact that there are basic physiological and psychological differences between women and men. After all, how can women and men possibly eat the same way and expect to lose weight? It's not possible, yet other diet books use a "one diet fits all" philosophy. The result is that when we don't lose weight fast enough or we don't lose it at all or—worse yet—when we compare ourselves to others we know, we wonder why we're not successful. We then use our lack of success as an excuse to stop dieting.

Over the years, in my role as associate medical director of the Atkins Center for Complementary Medicine in New York City, I worked with thousands of people who were trying to diet. At the center, everyone was placed on the same diet, with few variations. After years of experience, I saw that this was clearly not the way for everyone. There are differences in how a person metabolizes food, and the Atkins diet, as good as it was, did not take that into consideration at all.

Besides the differences between the sexes, there are also eating differences having to do with the stage of life you're in, which doesn't necessarily mean the same thing as your chronological age. Through my years of clinical practice, I have noticed certain stages of life that correspond to different dieting needs. There are four different female stages and three different male stages. So I subdivide *Thin For Good* into different categories according to your stage of life. One quiz for women and another for men will help you determine exactly in which stage you should start your diet. This is a critical issue, because just as every human being should not be on the same diet, every woman or man should not be on the same diet as women or men in different stages of life.

Another breakthrough is the diet I have devised for vegetarians—the first low-carbohydrate vegetarian diet available. So, even if you are lacto-ovo or a strict vegan, *Thin For Good* can help you lose weight the healthy way, too.

Included as part of the diet program are nutritional supplements. These are essential for any dieter. As there are so many to choose from and the array can be confusing, I have laid out a plan that covers the most common needs of any dieter. Individual supplement programs are outlined for both men and women, based on what stage of life you are in. This takes into account the most common health issues, such as menopause for women and prostate problems for men. The information found in this section will take the confusion out of a most difficult task.

With these concepts and tools, I believe that *Thin For Good* is the solution you need to break the previously inevitable cycle of yo-yo dieting.

When I was young I had no idea that I would be dedicating my life to nutritional medicine. I did know at an early age, however, that I wanted to help people lose weight. The reason was simple: I was an extremely overweight child and, over the years, I have been fortunate enough to learn that it is possible to lose weight forever.

After I initially lost my excess weight, I have never put it back on, yet I know firsthand what a lifelong struggle it can be—not so much to lose weight, but to keep it off. Many of my patients don't believe I was ever overweight (or simply "heavy," as my parents called it) because of my appearance today. But believe me, it's true.

In the years after medical school, I read every diet book I could find. Two problems all of them shared were 1) the inability to describe a proper maintenance program—the most essential component of any dietary regime, as far as I am concerned, and 2) the lack of a psychological game plan. After all, how can anyone lose weight without a practical program, with both a nutritional and a mind-body perspective, for how to change improper eating habits and, most importantly, a roadmap for how to learn new habits?

The patients I have treated—first at the Atkins Center and now at the Centers for Integrative and Complementary Medicine—have almost always been successful because I am able to modify their diet in order to make it work for them. My secret is to individualize each patient's program by using many of the methods you are about to read. *Thin For Good* will provide you with many of the tricks I learned to get even the most stubborn body to lose weight.

The emphasis needs to be on teaching you how to lose weight and be successful for a lifetime—not only for the first few weeks.

With *Thin For Good*, you will not only enjoy the benefits of low-carbohydrate eating, but you will enjoy something stronger: the power of your mind working with you, not against you. This time, truly make it thin for good.

Let's get started!

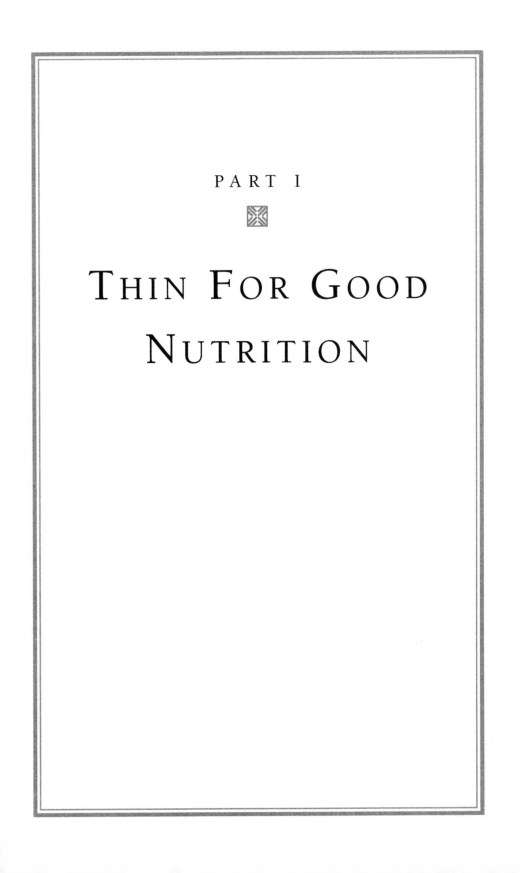

PART I

# THIN FOR GOOD
# NUTRITION

# CHAPTER 1

# Dieting and Your Emotions

## Food as Emotional Support

I wasn't always so thin. It seems like a lifetime ago, but I was once 60 pounds heavier than I am now. And, like most of us, deep down I know exactly how I got to be that way.

In my earlier years, before I lost weight, if the subject of dieting arose—and it often did—there was absolutely no support from my parents. To them, my two sisters and I did not have a problem. In fact, my parents encouraged us to eat—and if we didn't, they believed that something was wrong with us, that we must be ill. After all, it was the way they were raised—good Italian family values. Pasta wasn't the main course, it was simply a warm-up for the main course. Every meal was an adventure, and every meal had more than one course. Fortunately, in my teenage years, I was able to lose weight—much to the chagrin of my parents—and ultimately overcome the problem of obesity. At least up until now.

I say "up until now" because the struggle with weight is a lifelong battle, and to see it otherwise is a big mistake. For many of us, this struggle begins in childhood and never seems to end. Today, I look in the mirror and I still see that overweight child staring back at me. I believe I always will.

This does not mean, however, that I have to *be* that overweight child. I have made such a commitment to being thin that it takes precedence over almost anything else in my life.

Looking back, I realize that food was not mere sustenance. Rather, it became a substitute for many of life's emotional needs: love, happiness, support. Food was always there to comfort me when I was feeling down, and to cheer me up when things weren't going my way. I used food to soothe, to fill the empty places, to relieve disappointment. Feeling rejected? Eat. Feeling disappointed? Eat. Feeling sad? Eat. What a bunch of baloney! This was a learned response to food, and something I needed to change if I was ever going to stay thin for good.

Only now do I know that food is just that—food. This is the first mind-body concept I want you to understand: Food is what you eat, what your body needs to survive. Nothing more. Don't give it any other meaning in your life than that. An easy concept to see, but a more difficult one to live.

Repeat after me: Food is only meant to be nourishment. Food is what our bodies need in order to function. Food will never marry me, food will never make me rich, food will never give me all that I desire, and food will never make me truly happy. Saying it is the easy part. Now we have to put it into practice.

## An Exercise: What Does the Word "Diet" Mean to You?

One of the biggest problems people have with losing weight is that they don't understand what the word "diet" means. After you finish reading this paragraph, write down in each space provided one word that tells what "diet" means to you, or how dieting makes you feel. No reading ahead. GO!

1. _____      2. _____

3. _____      4. _____

If you wrote "deprivation," or some other word that has a similar meaning, you are thinking the same way I did for so long.

The word "diet" does not mean deprivation. It simply means "a way of eating," or what you eat. For instance, there is a high-protein diet, a vegetarian diet, or a high-carbohydrate diet, and many variations in between. The word "diet" describes the type of foods that are primarily consumed. That's it. Deprivation is simply not part of the equation, and cannot become a part of the equation if you are to be successful. Diet has no beginning and no end.

You are the one who makes it mean deprivation, in the same way that it is you who makes yourself believe that food is going to satisfy your emotional needs by making you feel better. *Thin For Good* will help change this behavior.

### Stop the Cravings for Good

How often have you been overtaken by food cravings when you are dieting? Lots of times, I'd bet. Our emotions seem to take control of us. In order to be a successful dieter, you are going to learn how to control these cravings with the mind-body medicines I provide later in the book. Food cravings will no longer control you; it will be the other way around. For the first time in your life, probably, you are going to take control over these food cravings, and you are going to be a happy dieter because of it.

Do you ever feel better immediately while you're eating a food that you know isn't good for you and then feel ten times worse right afterward—either because you're too stuffed, or because you feel so guilty about having eaten the food you didn't want to eat, or because you knew it was bad for you? I know I do. *Thin For Good* will teach you to stop that negative feeling from happening.

## The Secret of Mind Over Calories

I believe that what has made me a successful dieter and made many of my patients successful is the Mind Over Calories concept that I have developed. I have come up with a set of phrases, which I call mind-body medicines, that helps me live life as a thinner person. I have developed these over the past decade and I am happy to be able to share them with you.

I have found that Mind Over Calories is beneficial not only to those who are in the midst of the *Thin For Good* initiation diet, but also in the forever phase. In this book I have included a series of thirty phrases, or reminders, that will help you get through each of the first thirty days of this new diet plan. In chapter 21, I provide many more. The most meaningful ones for you should be repeated throughout your life, as I do, to help maintain your weight.

## The Eleven Emotional Levels of Eating

At the end of each of the first eleven chapters, I am going to explore a different emotion that plays a key role in dieting. Please read each level even if the particular chapter does not apply to you. I have found that there are distinct emotional stages when it comes to dieting. Over the years, I have observed that many of my patients move through these emotions during their weight loss process. Many get stuck in one particular phase or another, too. However, when you are able to acknowledge that these stages exist and are able to work through them, that is when you have the highest chance for lifelong success. Many of us have fought hard to ignore these emotions, thinking they will simply disappear when we reach our target weight. They don't, and it's truly harmful to think they will. There can be no true success without that admission.

I will include at the end of the discussion of each emotion the mind-body medicines that are most helpful in dealing with that particular emotion. For the first time, you will be able to enlist the help of something other than the actual mechanics of a weight-loss diet to achieve your goal.

Learning to handle these emotions in a positive way is the most beneficial thing you can ever do, and not only with respect to dieting. The understanding of these emotions and the mind-body techniques offered in this book will have a lasting impact on your life. You will learn to release or transform the negative emotions and learn to live with the positive ones. This may seem like a difficult concept now, but by the end of the book I can guarantee that it will seem like second nature—and you will be yet another success story.

## THE ELEVEN EMOTIONAL LEVELS OF EATING
# LEVEL 1: ANGER

Anger is the emotion most of us experience when we begin our diets. We are angry with the way we look and the way we feel. We may even be angry with the world, thinking life has dealt us a bad hand. Sometimes we express this emotion as disgust, or a feeling of not being able to take it anymore. Why shouldn't we be angry? We are overweight or we are unhealthy or both. No matter how we individually express this emotion, it all boils down to the same thing—anger.

You must understand that this is a normal response and probably universal to being overweight. However, it needn't be a completely negative emotion. After all, it has brought you to wanting to start a diet, hasn't it?

In an attempt to get to the bottom of this anger, I often have patients write down the answers to some simple questions to help define where exactly this emotion is coming from.

1. What makes me really mad?
2. What don't I like about myself?
3. What don't I like about my job?
4. What don't I like about my spouse/significant other?
5. What do I resent about others?

### Bonus Question: Why do I feel this way?

The real key to understanding and dealing with your anger is to answer the question of why you feel this way. However, answering the *what* questions will go a long way toward helping you understand why you may be angry at being overweight or unhealthy.

### Mind-Body Medicines That May Help With Anger
- Remember Mind Over Calories
- Make a commitment to being thinner.
- Ego is our only limitation in our quest for better health.

### Recipes That May Help with Anger (see chapter 22)
- Stuffed Mushrooms
- Lemon Cheesecake Squares

# CHAPTER 2

⊠

# Carbs and Glucose

Jennifer, forty-two, visited my office because she wanted to lose 20 pounds. Like many women, she had gained those pounds gradually, in the years after she graduated from college, and especially after the birth of her first child. Over this period, she was getting less exercise, primarily because, with all the responsibilities that came with child-rearing and a career, there was less and less time to work out or to do anything more physical than getting in and out of her car. She did admit to having several exercise machines at home, but she never bothered to use them anymore. She told me that she had not significantly changed the amount of food she ate. In fact, she believed she was eating "healthier." Jennifer was getting a little fed up with the whole dieting yo-yo. She couldn't understand how eating healthier was making her heavier.

The first thing I did after my initial interview with Jennifer was review her food diary—something each of my patients completes, which lists everything that goes into their mouths. I needed to know exactly what she was eating and what she considered healthy so I could try to figure out ways to change the way she dealt with food.

I placed Jennifer on the Thin For Good initiation phase specifically formulated for a woman in her stage of life: the perimenopausal/menopausal woman. I also explained the mind-body medicines so integral to my program. She immediately loved this part of the diet because she knew that unless her head was wrapped around a new idea, she was never going to follow through. Although her periods were still regular, Jennifer did not know that a woman's hormones and metabolism begin to change about ten years before her period stops.

Within two weeks on the program, Jennifer had lost 6 pounds. She was ecstatic, as this was the first diet in a long time that enabled her to lose any weight at all. She studied her mind-body exercises with fervor and was amazed at how they made the entire dieting process that much easier. Within three months, Jennifer had lost the entire 20 pounds.

To some, this may seem like a slow process, but slow progress is better than no progress at all. Remember, Jennifer had been having difficulty losing any weight and she thought she was on a healthy diet. I told this to Jennifer and I tell it to you: *It is important to keep in mind that we don't get overweight overnight* (it only seems that way), *so it may take some time to lose weight.* Be patient. Don't let yourself get discouraged easily.

## Keep a Diet Diary

You probably already know what diet diaries are. I'd like to review Jennifer's diary with you, and I think you will be amazed at what was in it. You'll recall that Jennifer told me she was eating healthier than ever before and yet she was gaining weight. When I asked Jennifer what she liked to eat, she proudly replied, "I eat a healthy diet, you know, cereal with bananas or a bagel for breakfast; yogurt for lunch; and a light pasta dish for dinner."

Although Jennifer believed this was a healthy diet, I knew otherwise. I can't even say I was surprised, since this kind of supposedly healthy "diet" is one I need to change with my new patients almost every day.

Take a closer look at Jennifer's daily diet. Everything she ate had no fat, and yet she still managed to gain weight. The simple reason is that everything Jennifer ate either contained sugar or was sugar itself. No fat. Plenty of sugar. A gain of 20 pounds. You don't have to be Einstein to figure out what's wrong with this equation.

How frustrating this was for Jennifer! And how angry do you think this made her feel? She and countless others like you face this situation every day. You follow the rules. You do everything right. You make no mistakes, and yet you still don't lose a pound. How does this make you feel? I have a pretty good idea, since I'm angry right now just writing this paragraph.

## The Dangers of Low-Fat, High-Carbohydrate Diets

The low-fat, high-carbohydrate diet that is currently in vogue in the mainstream medical community has rarely been tested in a group of individuals. In fact, when a low-fat diet was tested in a recent study in which individuals kept their dietary fat intake below 30 percent, it was found to actually increase an individual's risk of cardiac disease, not lower it.

The "low-fat myth" has been allowed to perpetuate to the point where the public believes that they can eat as many carbohydrates as they wish, just so long as the foods don't contain fat or cholesterol. This is a dangerous belief, and one that is making us fatter.

## The Carbohydrate-Triglyceride Link

Your body will produce cholesterol whether you eat any or not. Cholesterol plays a vital role in helping your body maintain good health. Cholesterol is found in every cell in your body, and your cells would fall apart if there were no cholesterol. No matter how much cholesterol you eat, your body will eliminate what it doesn't need through your bowels, unless you are also consuming too many other nutrients.

The real culprit is the typical North American diet. We consume too much of *everything*, thereby overwhelming our body's ability to eliminate what we don't need. Our bodies have a natural protective mechanism that allows us to store the excess food we consume, only to use it as needed during periods of starvation. This was an important tool thousands of years ago, but hardly needed today, at least in most parts of the Western world.

When we consume more carbohydrates than can be stored in the liver and muscles, or more than our body needs for brain power, these carbohydrates are converted to glucose. The body stores three of these molecules together as a more efficient way of storing the excess energy, as triglycerides (tri means "three"). Triglycerides are also stored in fatty tissue called adipose.

These excess triglycerides are what clog up the arteries. This is why it is probably more dangerous to have high levels of triglycerides than it is to have high levels of cholesterol. High levels of triglycerides lead to a higher incidence of heart disease and stroke.

Frustration leads to a lifetime of cravings and a feeling of never being fulfilled. It is not logical to think that most of us can live on a diet when we consume less than 20 percent of our calories in fat. Where's the joy in that? How satisfied are you going to feel eating this way for a lifetime? Most foods that have flavor also contain some fat. There are simply too many temptations and too many health benefits in healthy fats to deprive yourself for a lifetime of this major component of the food chain. In order for a diet to be successful, it has to be sustainable and enjoyable over the long haul.

## Food Was Her Obsession

Joan, fifty-one, visited my office because she was feeling increasingly fatigued. She found it increasingly difficult to make it through a work day without nodding off. She was also becoming increasingly focused on food. She needed to know exactly when her next meal was and, if it wasn't soon enough, if there would be ample time for snacking between her meals. Food, which Joan almost never thought about before, was suddenly becoming an obsession.

These feelings of fatigue and hunger crept up on Joan slowly throughout the day. She woke up each morning feeling fine and full of pep, but by about three o'clock in the afternoon, a couple of hours after lunch, her energy became completely sapped and she felt the need to take a nap. Unfortunately, because of the nature of her job, a midday nap was not possible. So

Joan pushed herself through this part of the day by eating some candy or having a couple of cups of coffee.

Joan was also experiencing an overwhelming sense of anxiety and irritability. Her moods seemed to change constantly throughout the day. One minute she was happy, the next she was angry. If she had to put her finger on it, she would say that her mood worsened when she was hungry, or almost always a few hours after eating. If she didn't snack, she felt as if she would rip someone's head off. She felt as if she were going through the worst part of her "changes" again, and she had no desire to experience that all over again.

After taking a comprehensive history and physical, I examined Joan's exhaustive food diary. She was meticulous in her detail and, not surprisingly, I immediately saw that she was consuming far too many high-carbohydrate, fat-free meals. Eating fat-free had become another obsession with her. She consumed nothing unless the label read "fat free." However, the amounts of the foods she ate was irrelevant to her; after all, the foods she was eating were fat-free and therefore, she reasoned, quantity didn't matter.

Was she ever wrong! Joan had begun to gain weight and she simply chalked it up to all the things she had heard from her friends about the change of life. She thought it was perfectly natural for a woman to add a few pounds during and after menopause. This is a common misconception. She was miserable and quite moody. She was also starting to get really angry and was finding it difficult to control her rage, especially in the afternoons when she felt her worst.

## Sugar and Emotions

During Joan's medical testing, I performed a glucose tolerance test, which in her case was abnormal. In the third hour of the administration of the glucose, Joan's blood sugar dropped to a low of 45, whereas the normal low should be about 65. By the same token, her second hour insulin level was 172 units. The absolute highest this level should ever be and still be within the normal range is 60. This simple test was able to tell me exactly why Joan felt the way she did after eating.

When blood sugar drops to such low levels, a few of the symptoms a person can experience include irritability, anxiety, restlessness, sleepiness, and unclear thinking. Joan's fatigue was simply the very common result of her low blood sugar, or hypoglycemia, brought on by her fat-free, high-carbohydrate diet. As a result of her diet, Joan was consuming more sugar in one day than I eat in an entire month.

Most people aren't aware of the fact that most fat-free foods contain added sugar. This is done for a reason; when fat is removed from a food, something must be added in order for the food to retain some flavor. Also, fat adds consistency to food, and once the fat is removed, sugar must be added to take its place; otherwise the food would fall apart. When was the last time you thought about how much extra sugar there was in a food that didn't contain any fat? I'd bet it wasn't even a consideration.

I have found that many people experience these daily mood swings before they come to see me. All they need to do is to regulate their blood sugar better by eating a proper diet. This may eliminate most people's moodiness within a few days. If not eliminated completely, almost always the moodiness is better under control.

I placed Joan on the initiation phase of the Thin For Good program for women of her stage and within a week those afternoon slumps were gone, her moods had improved, and she had shed 5 pounds. I also gave her the mind-body medicines. She found these to be incredibly useful, especially when she was craving certain things, or when frustration at work sent her looking for something sweet. She was surprised at how important these exercises became to her. They made her realize the role food played in her life and how it needed to change if she ever wanted to keep the weight off, and always feel this good.

She was really doing well. By the end of a month, 15 pounds were gone and she had more energy than she had had since she was in her twenties. And, of course, she continued with the mind-body exercises as she considered them the main reason she was able to stick with this plan rather than giving up, as she had done on so many other diets in the past.

## Men Have Trouble Metabolizing Sugar, Too

Harvey, a thirty-two-year-old body builder, appeared in my office one day because, for the first time in his life, he was developing a slight belly. The "six-pack" stomach he had worked on so hard for most of his adult life was disappearing. He was still working out five days a week, lifting weights as well as doing some form of aerobic exercise. Yet, his belly (as he called it) continued to grow slowly larger, to the point where his waist had grown to 34 inches from the trim 31 inches that he had maintained most of his life. He needed to lose about 30 pounds.

Harvey was confused, because despite his growing waist, the rest of his body was remaining the same. What made it even more mysterious to Harvey was that he wasn't eating any more than he had, nor any differently, and he certainly was not exercising any less. He was beginning to chalk it all up to simply getting older, when a friend of his recommended he come to see me.

After reviewing Harvey's blood work, I went over the results of his glucose tolerance test with him. Before I even saw the figures, I knew that he was going to have an abnormal result because a classic sign of someone who has trouble metabolizing sugar is growth around the midsection without an appreciable increase in size anywhere else on the body.

Over the course of the five-hour test, Harvey's blood sugar rose from a normal starting point to a number somewhat higher than normal, then quite slowly fell back into the normal range, without ever falling into the hypoglycemic range. His insulin levels were markedly elevated to three times the normal amount. No wonder he was having trouble losing weight. Insulin is a storage hormone and when your body secretes too much insulin it will cause your body to store weight.

I explained to Harvey that he had to eliminate all the simple carbohydrates—including all sugars—from his diet, stop the carbohydrate-loading cycle, and eat more fats. He was flabbergasted, because this advice flew in the face of the prevailing wisdom. How was he going to be able to eat out with friends? What would they think? I also told him that I was going to put him on a diet specifically for men and he readily agreed.

The hardest thing to discuss with him was the mind-body part of the program. I often find this to be the most difficult part for men to think that they need. Once they read it through, though, and see how it can help, the trepidation vanishes.

Once Harvey took my advice, the results were incredible. Within two weeks, he lost 12 pounds, and his "six-pack" returned within four weeks. The first thing he attributed this success to was the mind-body medicines. He couldn't believe he was saying that, but he was quite serious. He used them to learn how to be social and still be dieting. I was thrilled. Harvey also reported that he was having some of the best workouts of his life. He was filled with energy and better able to work out longer. Within two months, Harvey had lost the entire 30 pounds he wanted to, and he was sending all his friends to my office because they were amazed by the results he was able to obtain.

## The Many Faces of Sugar

Most people don't realize the implication the results of the glucose tolerance test may have on their health. Despite what your conventional medical doctor may tell you, it is an incredibly valuable test. Briefly, the glucose tolerance test checks your body's ability to process sugar and sugarlike substances. Remember, sugar comes in many disguises, such as:

- brown sugar
- corn syrup
- high-fructose corn syrup
- maple syrup
- dextrin
- raw sugar
- fructose
- honey
- molasses
- polyols
- dextrose
- hydrogenated starch
- galactose
- glucose

- invert sugar
- sorbitol
- fruit juice concentrate
- lactose
- sorghum

- maltose
- mannitol
- turbinado sugar
- xylitol
- sucrose

And this list does not include some of the many other guises sugar takes such as pasta, white bread, bagels, pretzels, soda, and fruit juice itself, to name a few. All of these products are metabolized by the body as sugar, with only minimal differences. Your body has no way of knowing the source of the sugar; it just knows that it is there, and that it must be metabolized, and therefore, the body must secrete insulin.

Insulin plays an important role by lowering blood glucose levels. Insulin accomplishes this because it is the body's main storage hormone—its role is to put aside excess carbohydrate calories in the form of fat. The body is directed by insulin not only to store these extra carbohydrates as fat, but also not to release any of the stored fat. Consequently, insulin is known as a locking hormone.

With this in mind, how can a diet that is high in carbohydrates—and therefore high in insulin secretion by its very nature—possibly cause an overweight person to lose weight?

## The Glucose Tolerance Test Explained

In the glucose tolerance test, or GTT (a test I consider critical to treating a patient), you are given a certain amount of sugar, based on your body weight, and then your blood is taken at hourly intervals until the end of the test. The test generally runs for about five to six hours.

From the results of this test, I can tell whether or not a patient is predisposed to coronary artery disease, hypercholesterolemia (high cholesterol), hypertriglyceridemia (high triglycerides), type II diabetes, or hypoglycemia. I'll even be able to tell whether or not the person will have difficulty losing weight, because correcting how sugar is metabolized is the key to success.

I also examine insulin levels, which are obtained by another blood test taken while fasting and again two hours after eating sugar. With this information, I can then design a diet that will work for the individual patient, with relative certainty that it will succeed. The proper regulation and balance of insulin levels and how sugar is metabolized is the true bottom line of health, and that is precisely what my diet does for you.

Several researchers have linked dietary indiscretions, such as the overabundance of sugar, with coronary thrombosis, atherosclerosis, obesity, and platelet abnormalities, which may lead to stroke. Heavy sugar consumption causes insulin resistance. The most severe case of insulin resistance leads to type II diabetes.

However, there are more subtle forms of insulin resistance. They may not be severe enough to cause overt glucose disturbances and hence be classified as diabetes, but they may still be harmful to your health and cause more subtle changes in your glucose tolerance. There is no getting around the fact that aging is associated with insulin resistance. Many diseases that come along with aging, such as obesity, hypertension, and cardiovascular diseases, are related to this insulin problem.

Age-related insulin resistance does not lead to overt diabetes in most of us, yet it will lead to higher levels of glucose and higher levels of insulin in your bloodstream because of your body's inability to respond well to the insulin that is secreted. As you age, your body loses its ability to process insulin as well as it should.

## Understanding the Glycemic Index

In a diet such as the one I have used successfully with thousands of patients, one of the key ingredients is balance. *It is essential to balance how you eat foods.* Once you eliminate all the simple carbohydrates and sugars from your diet, then your body is able to secrete insulin the way nature intended, slowly throughout a meal.

A simple tool that may help you figure out what foods will slowly be metabolized by your body is the *glycemic index*, a scale that tells us how easily a particular food is metabolized into sugar, and how quickly it will be metabolized. A good rule of thumb is the higher the number, the more you should avoid that particular food. However, there are subtleties associated with the glycemic index. For example, fat will decrease a food's glycemic index, so ice cream has a low number. Yet you would want to avoid this food, especially when trying to lose weight! Use the glycemic index for whole foods and then the rule of thumb will apply.

The following table shows the glycemic index for some common foods. Note that alcohol is not included on this list because of testing inaccuracies. It is metabolized by the body as a simple carbohydrate and therefore it is assumed that it is close to 100, if not higher. For a complete listing, you can refer to several books exclusively on this topic.

### Some Common Foods and Their Glycemic Index*

| Food | Glycemic Index | Food | Glycemic Index |
|---|---|---|---|
| Puffed rice | 127 | French fries | 95 |
| Pretzels | 118 | Brown rice | 94 |
| Puffed rice cakes | 105 | Macaroni and cheese | 92 |
| Mashed potatoes | 104 | Carrots | 92 |
| White rice | 103 | Strawberry jam | 90 |
| White bread | 100 | Banana | 90 |

| Food | Glycemic Index | Food | Glycemic Index |
|------|----------------|------|----------------|
| Papaya | 90 | Milk | 49 |
| Corn | 90 | Hot chocolate | 49 |
| Parsnips | 87 | Apple | 45 |
| Mango | 85 | Broccoli | 45 |
| Apricot | 85 | Peanut butter | 40 |
| Peas | 75 | Pear | 40 |
| Pasta | 71 | Peach | 40 |
| Orange juice | 65 | Yogurt, plain | |
| Dark bread | 58–70 | unsweetened | 35 |
| Cookies | 54–98 | Beans, most | |
| Candy bar | 51–74 | varieties | 30–50 |
| Orange | 55 | Plum | 30 |
| | | Grapefruit | 25 |

*Adapted from Jenkins, et al., *American Journal of Clinical Nutrition*, 1981.

Since there are so many positive health benefits that can be obtained by eating in a way that regulates the insulin mechanism in your body, my diet is perfectly suited to help you not only lose weight, but also get healthy both physically and psychologically. And since insulin plays a strong role in the degeneration that is associated with aging, anything that decreases the secretion of insulin in your body will help to slow down your aging process.

## Healing Syndrome X

Phil, forty-two, came to my office because he was recently diagnosed with high blood pressure and told that he would have to remain on medication for the rest of his life. The side effect of the medication was a decrease in libido and ability to perform sexually, something Phil was not too happy about. Phil, a smoker, just 10 pounds overweight, was a weekend warrior who could always be found exercising in some way on the weekend, depending on the time of year.

The first thing I did was conduct a glucose tolerance test with insulin levels, as well as routine blood tests, a measurement of his cholesterol levels, including the good and the bad levels, and a homocysteine level. Not surprisingly, Phil's insulin levels were extremely elevated. His glucose tolerance test showed him to be markedly hypoglycemic. He had very high triglyceride levels of 375, an extremely low HDL level of 26 (the good cholesterol), and a normal homocysteine level.

After encouraging Phil to quit smoking, I placed him on the initiation phase of the diet that was correct for his stage of life. I also gave him some nutritional supplements and explained the mind-body medicines.

Phil performed admirably on the diet and was able to bring his blood pressure down in about eight weeks. His triglyceride levels fell precipitously (a good thing) and his HDL cholesterol increased markedly (another good thing). In large part because of the meditations I gave him, he was also able to quit smoking. He simply applied the concepts of what I was discussing to smoking instead of food, as he did not have a serious weight problem, and he was able to quit a two-pack-per-day habit.

Phil suffered from Syndrome X, a recently understood medical condition that is caused by insulin resistance and hyperinsulinemia (too much insulin in your blood) which leads to glucose intolerance, hypertriglyceridemia (high triglycerides), obesity, and hypertension. Now he's healthy again, simply by changing the way he eats.

## How to Stay Younger Longer

In some studies, it has been suggested that insulin resistance even plays a role in aging and tumor formation. I don't wish to get into a long discussion of the effect sugar has on cancer cells and on the possible formation of new cancer cells, but I do want to discuss its effects on the aging process, something most of us want to avoid as much as we can.

I don't pretend that the Thin For Good program is some kind of fountain of youth. You should not expect it to reverse the aging process so you look ten years younger than your chronological age, although that may happen. Instead, I am talking about trying to slow down some of the things that happen to us as we age, such as heart disease, diabetes, atherosclerosis, and cancer. Controlling these conditions could help slow down the aging process as we know it, and further prolong your life in the process.

The diet I include in this book will make your body a more efficient metabolizer of glucose by eliminating most of the sugar you would normally consume and giving your body more nutritionally dense foods. Simply put, manipulation of the diet by influencing the glucose/insulin system may favorably affect your life span and reduce the incidence of chronic disorders associated with aging.

Think about what this could mean. *More stamina, increased energy, better skin, stronger hair and nails, longer life span, better sex life, and better moods— all as a result of simply changing what you put in your mouth and how you think about and relate to food.*

Almost anyone can be successful on this diet plan. You simply need confidence, motivation, and the proper psychological tools—and of course you also need a diet plan you can live with. All of these things Thin For Good will give you.

# THE ELEVEN EMOTIONAL LEVELS OF EATING
## LEVEL 2: FRUSTRATION

Frustration has to be the most common emotion my patients have reported in the course of their program. It is the single most important emotion that I have had to overcome time and time again in my quest to remain thin. How could it not be? It's frustrating to see people who seem to be able to eat whatever they want and not gain weight. It's frustrating to see the people who eat whatever they want and do not seem to care about how they look or what they are doing to their arteries. And one of the toughest frustrations comes from knowing that you have done everything right on a diet and still can't lose any weight.

After the anger has set in and you have resolved to do something positive about your weight, frustration is usually the next emotion on the scene. This can be a very negative emotion, because it can be the main reason most people give up the fight. I want you to acknowledge that the frustration is real and that it is an almost universal emotion when it comes to dieting. Don't feel singled out. You are going to be comparing yourself only to yourself, and no one else. Let's use that frustration you have to melt the pounds away. As a result, that frustration will no longer be used against you. Instead, you are going to harness its power and you are going to lose weight.

You have every reason to feel the way you do. Now let's do something to change it into something a bit more positive by answering these questions:

1. What makes me frustrated?
2. Who makes me frustrated?
3. What would make things less frustrating for me?
4. Can I do anything about the situations in the answers to the above questions?
5. If the answer is no, does that make it more frustrating?

### Bonus Question: Is the frustration more about myself than about these other things?

This question is perhaps the most difficult to answer and will help you get to the bottom of the levels of frustration that you are experiencing. Frustration is all about different levels. No emotion is without those levels. We have to learn to make important distinctions and then know what we have the power to change and what we don't. It all comes down to what we can live with. It's time to get your house in order and learn how to live with certain food truths that may not be so comfortable for you.

Acknowledging the cause of the frustration can help change this into a tool that can help you, rather than hinder you. By clearing away your frustration and improving your self-esteem in the process, you may even improve your love life along the way!

**Daily Mind-Body Medicines That May Help with Frustration**
- Energy has no limitations in our drive for thinness.
- Don't let what is happening to you control how well you do on your diet.
- Work to change the negative dieting situation.

**Recipes That May Help with Frustration**
- Spinach and Ricotta Dumplings
- Korean Short Ribs

# CHAPTER 3

❧

# The Healing Power of Fats

Jim, forty-seven, came to my office because he was having second thoughts about his health. He had recently been to see his family doctor because he wanted to lose some weight and decrease his cholesterol. He was getting a little sluggish, did not have the same energy he'd had even five years ago, and on rare occasions found himself impotent. He was concerned because his father and two uncles had each had their first heart attack around the age of fifty. Since Jim was fast approaching this age, he did not want the same thing to happen to him, and he felt time was running out. Because of his family history and his own medical history, Jim was on high blood pressure medications and cholesterol reducing agents, and was taking an aspirin each day.

His doctor told him not to worry because he was only 15 pounds overweight, and if he wanted to lose some weight, he should just cut out all the fat he was eating. His doctor also increased the amount of his cholesterol-lowering medication because Jim's cholesterol, after three months on the drug, was still slightly elevated at 210; his HDL, or good cholesterol, was low at 38, and his triglyceride levels were a whopping 245.

Jim was unhappy with this advice, and I don't blame him. At most, Jim was in his doctor's office for five minutes after having waited close to two hours, and Jim felt that since he was faced with serious decisions, his doctor owed him more than just a few minutes of his time. The second thing that annoyed Jim was that the doctor told him to follow some low-fat diet. Jim felt that this kind of diet did not work for real men; real men need fat, was his contention. He knew he could never lose weight on a diet that was designed for his wife. Jim's reasoning was, "Women like lettuce and can be satisfied, men don't." Jim was getting a little angry because the advice he was getting was not working for him, and he wanted a plan that was going to be formulated with him in mind, not a plan that was formulated for everyone.

Not only did Jim know he could not stay on this low-fat diet, no matter how hard he tried, but he also knew that such a diet did nothing for his cholesterol numbers. In fact, a low-fat diet often made his numbers worse. His good cholesterol often went down, and his triglyceride number went up—the exact opposite of what we want to see happen. With this knowledge, at a friend's suggestion, Jim decided to try me.

I conducted a thorough history and physical examination, including routine blood tests and a glucose tolerance test. I also measured Jim's insulin levels, because it has been shown that high insulin levels, or hyperinsulinemia, play a role in heart disease.

Jim's glucose tolerance test was quite abnormal, falling to a low of 60 from a high of 199. His two-hour insulin level was 105 units. A normal two-hour insulin level would be no more than 60 units. A 140-point drop between the highest and lowest glucose level was also not good. The healthiest individuals have a range of 80 to 90 points maximum.

I explained the results of his tests to him and what they implied, and then I taught him the initiation phase of my Thin For Good diet. In a nutshell, this involved decreasing the amount of simple carbohydrates and sugars in his diet, increasing the amount of good fats and complex grains, and, ideally, increasing his amount of exercise and practicing the mind-body techniques.

Jim's reaction was, "You've got to be kidding, Doc! How could I eat that way and actually lower my risk for heart disease? Aren't fats bad for you?" After he got over the initial shock, he was quite pleased to see that this was a diet a man could stay on. None of those tiny portions to worry about. No stupid points to count. Just eating from the food groups that were allowable—that was something he could do. When he left my office, I could tell that he still wasn't convinced about all the mind-body stuff, but I hoped that he would try to incorporate it once I told him that it was an essential part of the key to his success, and that getting off the medication would probably restore a normal sex life. That's all he had to hear to at least guarantee me he would give it a shot.

Within six weeks, Jim had lost 16 pounds, his triglyceride level had dropped 200 points to 45, his total cholesterol level dropped to 186, and his HDL, or good cholesterol, level increased to 52. And do you know what he thought was the best thing about the diet, other than the fact that it was specifically for men? He loved writing down all the mind-body medicines on index cards and carrying the message wherever he went. He never shared them with anyone but he would recite them and think about the message in the car and at night before he went to sleep. He found that one needed to do more than just say them. You had to feel them and know the meaning. He was shocked.

## Fat Can Be Good for You

As hard as it might be to believe, the majority of doctors never study nutrition. Consequently, based on their lack of information, I think it is at best unwise and at worst irresponsible of them to be giving patients nutritional advice.

Low-fat, high-carbohydrate diets can cause sharp decreases in the level of the desirable HDL cholesterol, and unfavorable increases in the levels of triglycerides, which was illustrated in Jim's case. In fact, HDL levels will more likely rise when good fatty acids, like olive oil, are introduced to the diet, and triglyceride levels will decrease when simple sugars and simple carbohydrates are eliminated from the diet.

Trans fatty acids, along with sugar, are the worst dietary offenders. Trans fatty acids are found in most processed foods in your kitchen cabinet and on grocery store shelves. These products include breads, cakes, cookies, and all fast or convenience foods. In short, many foods that are prepackaged likely contain trans fats. Trans fatty acids are the types of fat that result from the hydrogenation process used to lengthen the shelf life of common oils. In a later chapter, I'll teach you how to read food labels to avoid such things, and what to really look out for when shopping in the grocery store.

## Fats, Cravings, and Mood Swings

What we have been told about fats for so long is not true. We are constantly told that one thing is good for us and another is bad, only to receive the exact opposite news two weeks later. What are we to believe? No wonder you feel frustrated, angry, and even depressed. I can only tell you of the program that I have developed and the amazing health benefits that I have seen.

Studies have shown that the amount of fat you eat has no bearing on your risk of getting prostate or breast cancer. Studies have also shown that eating certain fats may decrease the incidence of certain types of cancer, decrease your chance of getting a stroke, make your menopause easier, make you happier, increase your memory and attention span, and make you feel better overall, not worse, as is commonly believed.

Did you know that the right types of fat may also play a role in moods and mood swings? This is because fat can help regulate your blood sugar. Fat takes longer for your body to digest, thereby slowing the release of blood sugar and hence insulin into your bloodstream, helping your metabolism operate more efficiently. This will absolutely help to lessen the severity of your mood swings, especially if they are diet related. Also, when dieting, fat will send a signal to your brain that you are full, helping you control food cravings and hunger.

Fat plays an extremely important role in the chemistry of your brain. Your brain is more than 60 percent fat, and low-fat diets deprive your brain of the essential fatty acids so vital to brain function. Is it any wonder that you feel depressed and experience brain fog on a low-fat diet? You are literally starving your brain of the nutrients it needs.

When you also add in the fact that fatty acids play a critical role in the control of inflammation, then the proper balance of fatty acids in our diets seems not only important in maintaining proper health, but critical to it.

It has been reported that the right balance of these fatty acids can help with learning difficulties, developmental delays, autism, and behavioral problems in kids; and mood disorders, memory difficulties, seizures, strokes, and other brain-related disorders in adults. Multiple sclerosis (MS) is a disease that destroys the myelin sheath that protects our nerves. This sheath is composed mostly of omega-3 fatty acids, a nutrient particularly lacking in the common American diet. Studies have shown that individuals with lower levels of omega-3 fatty acids also had more symptoms of attention deficit disorder and hyperactivity.

These fatty acids may even help to manage stress—who couldn't use that? Omega-3 fatty acids also help to control some of the negative actions of the omega-6 fatty acids. It all comes down to balance. If these fatty acids were properly balanced, as they are in my diet, there would most likely be less chronic disease.

## Think Like a Thin Person

Irene, forty-two, came to see me in a last-ditch effort to lose weight. She was totally disgusted because she had been religiously following the latest diet that she believed would help her lose weight. Over the years, she had been on a number of different diets and had followed every one of them to the letter. Initially, they worked and she would lose weight, but inevitably she would reach a plateau, get disgusted, go back to her old eating habits, and regain all the weight she had lost and then some. On some diets, she wouldn't lose weight at all, or she would lose weight but then throw in the towel because she found the diet too restrictive to maintain. Irene needed to lose about 100 pounds. She was also concerned because she was having elevated blood pressure readings for the first time in her life.

The diets that completely failed Irene were the typical low-fat, high-carbohydrate diets that allow you to count points while eating any food you want to or the ones with set meal plans. Following these diets, Irene found herself constantly hungry. She also found that when she was allowed to eat anything she wanted, so long as she stayed within a given point system, it was not helping her achieve her real goal, which was to establish long-term changes in her eating patterns so that she could get off the diet roller-coaster.

She had also tried the other low-carbohydrate, high-protein diets that allowed as much protein as she wanted, and found that she had no ability to control the amount of food she consumed, so that type of diet wasn't right for her either. She felt that these unlimited protein diets were great for men, but could never work for most women. She longed for a diet that could help her get through the rough times, while still being allowed to enjoy eating.

Irene resisted my diet for two reasons. The first reason was that she found eating protein far too restrictive. She thought that she would not be able to go out with the girls and eat what they were eating, and she found it to be a rather boring way to eat. The second reason was that she did not want a diet that encouraged unlimited amounts of anything. This was not going to do her any good because she already had the unlimited-amounts-of-food thing down to a science. It was not a successful way of eating for her, and it only made her heavier.

I explained that this is where my low-carbohydrate diet differs from some of the others. I don't allow unlimited portions of anything. What Irene needed was a new nutritional lifestyle program—one developed with women in mind, and one that could teach her how to think like a thin person. There is no denying that thin people think differently from the way we do. In my diet you are going to learn how to think like a thin person, or at the very least, learn how to get thinner.

I asked several more questions in our interview. Irene admitted that losing weight was becoming increasingly more difficult and that on her last attempt at dieting she had the hardest time she could ever remember. What made this so disturbing was that it was a diet on which she had been very successful in the past.

## Syndrome W

The fact that Irene was having so much trouble losing weight was not unusual, given her stage of life. Irene was in the perimenopausal stage of life. Menopause is something that lasts for years in most women. The changes that take place in a woman's body occur very gradually and long before the first recognizable symptom of menopause appears.

Medical science has just come up with a new term to describe women like Irene: syndrome W. These are people who start to gain weight in midlife, with weight gains greater than 20 pounds. The weight is concentrated around the abdomen and the hips, with an increase in waist measurement of more than 2 inches. People with this syndrome tend to binge eat, and have mildly elevated blood pressure.

When I explained the principles of my diet to Irene, she liked the fact that at last there was a diet that specifically addressed her issues. Other diets had not taken into account the differences in people at various stages of life. In fact, no other diets she had tried even took into account the differences between men and women and how their bodies handle dieting differently.

The diet plan I will outline in this book and the one that I outlined for Irene are life-stage and gender specific. Her diet plan allowed her to have some complex carbohydrates, which made it possible for her to stay on the diet without feeling deprived, which she had not been able to do on other low-carbohydrate diets that were always too restrictive in this category. And she could have them at most meals, not just at one meal or another. Furthermore, the diet regulated her food cravings so that after the first three days of this new plan, she had tremendous energy and had no food cravings of any kind. Her mood improved. By balancing the types of foods Irene ate, she was able to follow the diet so well that she lost 15 pounds in two weeks and the 100 pounds that was her ultimate goal in a mere thirteen months. Irene's blood pressure went down to normal after the first two months of the diet. Irene loved her daily mind-body medicines. She even taught me some of her own. She admitted that she would never have been able to stay on a diet for thirteen months without some sort of plan that incorporated her psyche. Most other diets ignore the fact that you have a brain. Mine doesn't. Irene loved that this was the first intelligent diet that she had ever been on. Her brain got exercise, even if the rest of her often didn't.

## The Types of Fat

As you may know, there are three types of fats: saturated, monounsaturated, and polyunsaturated.

### Category I: Saturated Fats

At room temperature, most saturated fats are solids or semisolids, with the exception of the tropical oils, such as palm or coconut oil. Saturated fats are the types of fats found in most red meats and are the fats that have given red meat and tropical oils a bad reputation. Most conventional nutritionists will tell you to avoid this type of fat. I am going to tell you, as I told Irene, that this should not be the case. In fact, there are many advantages to these types of fats and oils.

The tropical oils are antifungal and antibacterial. Two thirds of the saturated fats found in these oils are the short- and medium-chain fatty acids, which are healthy. Lauric acid, one such medium-chain fatty acid, is found in coconut oil and is also found in large quantities in human breast milk.

In red meat and in some dairy products there is a saturated fatty acid known as conjugated linoleic acid (CLA). Recent studies in animals have shown that high doses of this fatty acid may actually prevent some cancers, prevent heart disease, boost the immune system, and decrease body fat. Many body builders use this fatty acid in pill form in the belief that it will help them get more defined muscles. I have used it for patients who are having difficulty losing weight. Sometimes CLA can actually help increase the speed of your metabolism, which is useful when trying to lose weight.

## Category II: Monounsaturated Fats

Examples of monounsaturated fats are olive oil and canola oil. I am the biggest proponent of olive oil and one of the most vocal opponents of canola oil—when it is heated. Canola oil is made in Canada from the rapeseed, another in a long line of agricultural by-products that can be unhealthy for us. It is very high in omega-9 fatty acids, which makes it a good oil to use COLD. Once heated, it becomes extremely unstable and releases trans fatty acids, which may be even more dangerous than the trans fatty acids found in margarine. *So, to be clear, use canola oil cold, such as in salad dressings, but don't cook with it.*

Olive oil is the most benign of oils, and my oil of choice. It contains 80 percent monounsaturated fatty acids, and it is almost completely neutral in that it contains mostly omega-9 fatty acids that don't easily turn rancid when heated. Of course, some olive oils are better than others. I recommend looking for those that are cold-pressed, dark green, and offered in dark containers. Once you've purchased the olive oil, it should be stored away from the light in a cool area.

## Category III: Polyunsaturated Fats

The polyunsaturated oils you are most likely to be familiar with are corn, safflower, soybean, cottonseed, sunflower, peanut, walnut, fish, and flaxseed oils. All of these oils, however, are not created equal. One characteristic that separates the oils is the ratio of omega-6 to omega-3 fatty acids.

These two polyunsaturated fats, omega-6 and omega-3 fatty acids, are considered essential because they cannot be produced by the body and must be taken in through the diet. Omega-6 is known as alpha-linoleic acid. Omega-3 is known as alpha-linolenic acid.

The omega-3 fatty acid family is comprised of eicosapentanoic acid (EPA) and docosahexanoic acid (DHA). The omega-6 fatty acid family contains gamma-linolenic acid (GLA) and arachidonic acid (AA). These two fatty acids play major roles in our health, and the amount you eat is believed to have an influence on many of the chronic diseases we have become prone to.

The typical American diet is overloaded with omega-6 fatty acids, as they are found in most processed foods as well as in most fast foods and fried foods—a significant part of most Americans' diets.

# Balance Your Fatty Acids

Many researchers believe that people with diets high in omega-6 fatty acids suffer from higher levels of inflammation, which may eventually lead to such chronic conditions as asthma, allergies, arthritis, psoriasis, and colitis, to name just a few. Does this sound like anyone you know? I don't think there is a single one of us who has not suffered or does not currently suffer from one of these disorders. The imbalance occurs because our diets typically lack enough omega-3 fatty acids, and are too high in omega-6 fatty acids.

The omega-3 fatty acid family seems to promote better health by decreasing the level of inflammation found in your body, thereby decreasing your perception of pain. These fatty acids are believed to positively affect blood pressure, boost your immune system, and decrease the incidence of heart disease by making platelets less likely to clump together, thereby decreasing the chance of blood clots and stroke. They may also have a cholesterol-lowering effect, while improving cholesterol ratios (the good cholesterol rises and the bad cholesterol lowers). Omega-3 fatty acids are found in foods such as flaxseeds; cold saltwater fatty fish like mackerel, tuna, herring, cod, sardines, and salmon; walnuts; and some beans. The omega-3s can also be found in eggs that have been enhanced with these fatty acids.

Certain fats are indeed good for you and I've compiled a list so you can know which are the ones to avoid and which are the ones you should feed your family. I have rated these with gold, bronze, and lead medals. No oil deserves the silver medal as there is a big difference between the gold oils and the bronze ones.

---

### Gold Medal

*Use as you like.*

| | |
|---|---|
| Olive Oil: the gold standard for cooking | Coconut Oil |
| Flaxseed Oil (cold only) | Macadamia Nut Oil |
| Evening Primrose Oil (cold only) | Walnut Oil |
| Palm Oil | Canola Oil (cold only) |

### Bronze Medal

*Use sparingly because they contain a high proportion of omega-6 fatty acids. If you do use them, use them cold. Do not heat these oils; sparingly if you do.*

| | |
|---|---|
| Peanut Oil | Corn Oil |
| Sesame Oil | Soybean Oil |
| Safflower Oil | Cottonseed Oil |

### Lead Medal

*These should be avoided at all costs.*

| | |
|---|---|
| Canola Oil (when heated) | Margarine |

## How to Choose the Proper Cooking Oil

1. Use oil from a whole source, such as olives or fish.
2. Organic oils are preferable because they are free of chemicals.
3. Store your oil carefully, out of the light and in a cool dry place—even in the refrigerator.
4. Don't buy refined oils. These will say "refined" on the label.
5. Look for cold-pressed or expeller-pressed oils. This will mean that the oil was pressed at a lower temperature and therefore less likely to have spoiled.
6. If the oil tastes bitter, throw it away, as it has probably spoiled.

The real key to staying healthy through eating comes through dietary balance. The balance of fats in our diet is no exception. It is possible to eat fat and get thin. Not only is it possible, it is a necessity. There can be no successful diet program that does not balance what you eat while balancing the fatty acids you consume. There can be no successful maintenance program without that concept. The patients I've helped over the years are a testament to the proper balance.

# THE ELEVEN EMOTIONAL LEVELS OF EATING
## LEVEL 3: SADNESS

I place sadness third on the emotional continuum. This emotion doesn't usually set in until you have had the opportunity to experience the anger and frustration. It is an emotion that is usually very well hidden, in large part because most of us have made an attempt to cover it up at one point or another in our lives. After all, who has ever heard of an un-jolly fat person? Well, I have.

Many overweight people tend to overcompensate for being overweight by developing a razor-sharp wit, a great personality, or something else they hope will hide the fact that they are overweight. Eventually, this no longer works, and they must face the fact that being overweight makes them sad. This is not to say that every overweight person is sad. Far from it. There are overweight people quite content with their weight who have no desire to change. But I think you do.

Sadness is closely tied to feeling sorry for yourself. This is the way the majority of my patients express this emotion. They have made the commitment to change their way of life and their eating patterns, but once they do they begin to feel sorry for themselves, to mourn their old way of life. Some even blame the fact that they don't get to see old friends or acquaintances at their old haunts since they have changed their lifestyle because of their new commitment. Many tend to use this feeling of sadness as an excuse to give up the diet. Don't.

Let's look at this emotion more closely and see if you can make it work for you by asking yourself these simple questions:

1. What makes me feel sad?
2. What is making me feel this hurt?
3. What or who is making me feel unhappy?
4. What is making me feel disappointed?
5. Who is disappointing me?

### Bonus Question: What would make any of those things I just mentioned change my feeling of sadness to something else?

This is a tough question, because it makes you start wishing for things to happen that you may have no control over. This can return you to the previous emotional level—frustration. What I want you to do is try to figure out something you can do for yourself, something that is related only to you, in an attempt to make you feel a different emotion about each of your answers to the first five questions. Sadness doesn't have to be detrimental. It can teach us how to appreciate the power we have within ourselves to make ourselves happier, healthier, and in this case, thinner.

**Mind-Body Medicines to Help with Sadness**

- You will always be that overweight person.
- Realize the power of your thoughts and what you say about dieting.
- Our body creates a desire for the things we shouldn't have, especially when dieting.

**Recipes That May Help with Sadness**

- Chicken Licken
- Snickersnoo

# CHAPTER 4

# How to Read Labels and the New Food Pyramid

By the time you are finished reading this chapter, you will have more nutritional information than most physicians receive in their entire medical school training.

I used to host a radio program in New York City, and one of the most popular shows—one I was asked to do over and over—was the one in which I discussed food labels. So many people have questions about how to read food labels. It may seem simple but believe me, it isn't that easy. For instance, how do you know what you're reading when there are so many different words for the three basic macronutrients—protein, carbohydrate, and fat? What do the words actually mean? Is such-and-such really just another name for sugar? What's the difference between carbohydrates and fiber?

There are so many confusing words in the ingredient list that even I often have to look them up because, if I didn't, I'd be stumped when a patient asked me a question about them. But before we begin to dissect a food label and the ingredient list, let's begin with the basics.

## Food Label: A Primer Course

On page 37 is an actual food label for a breakfast cereal.

This label was taken from a typical breakfast product advertised as low in fat and sanctioned by the American Heart Association as "Heart Healthy." Now that you know the dangers of sugar, insulin, and heart disease, you should be able to tell me why "heart healthy" and this product should never be in the same sentence.

On a food label, the list of ingredients used in that product is required by law. These ingredients are listed in descending order by weight. The ingredient that weighs the least is shown last. Ingredients that make up 2 percent or less of a food by weight are listed at the end of the list in no particular order.

In the label of the low-fat diet food shown on the next page, the first ingredient is sugar, followed by two simple carbohydrates, corn meal and

## Nutrition Facts

Serving size: ¾ cup (30g)
Servings per package: About 13

| Amount per serving | ¾ cup cereal | cereal w/½ cup skim milk |
|---|---|---|
| **Calories** | 120 | 160 |
| Calories from fat | 10 | 10 |
| | **% Daily Value\*** | |
| **Total Fat** 1g | **1%** | **2%** |
| Saturated fat 0g | **0%** | **0%** |
| **Cholesterol** 0mg | **0%** | **0%** |
| **Sodium** 190mg | **8%** | **10%** |
| **Potassium** 50mg | **2%** | **7%** |
| **Total Carbohydrate** 27g | **9%** | **11%** |
| Sugars 14g | | |
| Other Carbohydrate 13g | | |
| **Protein** 1g | | |
| Vitamin A | 25% | 30% |
| Vitamin C | 25% | 25% |
| Calcium | 4% | 20% |
| Iron | 25% | 25% |
| Vitamin D | 10% | 20% |
| Thiamin | 25% | 25% |
| Riboflavin | 25% | 35% |
| Niacin | 25% | 25% |
| Vitamin B$_6$ | 25% | 25% |
| Folate | 25% | 25% |
| Vitamin B$_{12}$ | 25% | 25% |
| Phosphorus | 4% | 15% |

Not a significant source of Dietary Fiber.

% Recommended Daily Values based on:

| | Calories: | 2000 | 2500 |
|---|---|---|---|
| Total Fat | Less than | 65g | 80g |
| Sat. Fat | Less than | 20g | 25g |
| Cholesterol | Less than | 300mg | 300mg |
| Sodium | Less than | 2400mg | 2400mg |
| Potassium | | 3500mg | 3500mg |
| Total Carbohydrate | | 300mg | 375mg |
| Dietary Fiber | | 25mg | 30mg |

Calories per gram:
Fat: 9    Carbohydrate: 4    Protein: 4

**INGREDIENTS:** sugar, cornmeal, corn flour, corn syrup, modified corn starch, cocoa processed with alkali, wheat starch, partially hydrogenated soybean oil, salt, fructose, dionicium phosphate, beet powder and caramel color, baking soda, natural and artificial flavor, trisodium phosphate, sodium ascorbate (vitamin C), niacinamide (niacin), reduced iron, vitamin A (palmitate), pyridoxine hydrochloride (vitamin B$_6$), riboflavin (vitamin B$_2$), thiamin mononitrate (vitamin B$_1$), folic acid (folate), vitamin B$_{12}$ and vitamin D.

\*Based on a 2000-calorie diet

corn flour. The fourth ingredient is another sugar, corn syrup. The fifth, sixth, and seventh ingredients are more examples of simple carbohydrates; and the eighth ingredient is partially hydrogenated soybean oil.

Partially hydrogenated soybean oil is a trans fatty acid. It's not the soybean oil that is the problem, but the "partially hydrogenated" form that is the health risk here. This form of fat can be extremely dangerous to your health; it has been shown to lead to breast cancer and prostate cancer. And yet, this type of fatty acid does not need to be listed in the breakdown of the various types of fat on the food label. This is outrageous and an egregious error on the part of our government. If they are so interested in our consumption of fat, then the fat that is the most detrimental to our health should be listed so consumers can avoid it. The trouble is, trans fatty acids like these are present in almost every processed food product, a fact that the food industry wants to keep hidden as much as possible. A bill that would require this to be listed on food labels is currently being considered.

*Partially hydrogenated fat is the most unhealthy fat there is.* Since this fat is found in most store bought prepackaged foods, I would bet that you are consuming it on a daily basis.

I'd like you to put down this book right now, go into your kitchen cabinet and see just how many foods you own that have this ingredient. I predict you'll be shocked by how many there are. Partially hydrogenated fat should be the one food you try to avoid as often as you can. And you thought you were eating healthy!

The tenth ingredient in this product is sugar. So, in this heart-healthy, low-fat product, there are three forms of sugar: sugar itself, simple carbohydrates, and sugar in one of its many disguises. Suddenly, this ostensibly good-for-you product is beginning to look a lot less healthy, isn't it?

The other products on this list are flavorings, both artificial and natural, and the last ingredients are all the vitamins and natural preservatives that had to be replaced in this "heart-healthy, low-fat" food because of what was lost in the processing. Fortified foods are fortified because these nutrients have been lost when the food is processed. Take my advice: anytime you see foods that have been enriched for health reasons, stand clear, because there is a very good reason why these foods needed that enrichment. Nature provided us with foods that are actually nutritious. It is when people start to manipulate the food chain that problems arise.

After carefully reading the food label, you can see why I think this is such an unhealthy product. Yet many nutritional gurus in this country would endorse such a product, and countless others like this, simply because it is low in fat. Please don't let yourself be seduced by their rhetoric. Make healthy and informed decisions.

There are two other important things concerning food labels. First, look at the total amount of carbohydrates. This figure is broken down into total sugars, and either other carbohydrates or dietary fiber. If the sugars are greater than 10 percent of the total amount of carbohydrates, the product is very high in sugar and should be avoided, even when you reach the forever phase of the Thin For Good diet.

Second, see if the product is a significant source of dietary fiber. The jury is still out as to whether fiber is important in our diets, but one thing about fiber is certain: the higher the amount of fiber, the slower that food product will be absorbed into the bloodstream, keeping insulin levels on an even keel.

Fiber has been shown to have significant health benefits especially where your heart and cholesterol are concerned. This particular product is not a significant source of dietary fiber and says so right on the label. That is a definite sign for you to avoid this food.

My advice would be to memorize the salient points of this section on food labels, or better yet, photocopy it and take it to the grocery store with you so you will never mistakenly purchase something you think is healthy that isn't.

This primer on reading food labels should help you confidently go into a grocery store and make educated guesses about the health benefits or risks you face from any particular food. Even if you don't follow my diet for the rest of your life, this will be a valuable lesson that can apply to any diet you may follow in the future.

### What to Look For on Food Labels

1. Identify all the hidden sugars.
2. Identify all the not-so-hidden sugars.
3. Check the dietary fiber content.
4. Check for trans fatty acids—known as partially hydrogenated oils.
5. Check for total carbohydrates to total sugar—put the product back if the total is greater than 10 percent.
6. Look for the word "whole" when buying a grain product.
7. If you can't identify more than two of the ingredients in a food, don't buy it.
8. If there is more than one sugar source, don't buy it.

# The New and Improved Food Pyramid
## According to Dr. Fred

Originally, I developed this pyramid to teach parents why their children should be giving up sugar rather than fat, and incorporated it in my first book, *Feed Your Kids Well.* I used the concept of the pyramid because the USDA food pyramid is something that most kids are taught in school, and I wanted parents to have a readily available tool to teach their children the real way food is metabolized and how we process the food we eat. For this book, I am including this pyramid and a new one that I feel more accurately reflects how you should be eating.

## The Dieting Addict

Helen, thirty-seven, was a diet-addicted woman. She came to see me in an attempt to lose about 40 pounds. Even before walking into my office, she was completely convinced that she would never be able to do this on my diet. Helen was such a strong advocate of low-fat eating that she couldn't remember the last time she had eaten red meat, and more importantly, she couldn't conceive of being able to give up her bowls of pasta that she enjoyed at least four nights per week. They were, after all, fat free, and not only "healthy," but, she had been assured, eating them would help her to lose weight. The only reason she came to see me was that her sister had lost 75 pounds using my diet during the past year and, desperate to lose weight, she needed to see for herself what all the shouting was about.

The first thing I said to Helen was, "If a low-fat diet was so good for you, then how come you're 40 pounds overweight?" She explained that it was probably her fault as she found it hard to stick to her diet and was always craving sweets. She had no plan to mentally handle the challenges associated with dieting. In fact, she found herself to be constantly hungry. She didn't know what to do anymore, and was about to give up. She was looking for an answer, and I had one for her.

She was going through a divorce, she explained, and as a result she was using food as her solace. She felt terribly hungry all the time and, try as she might, she just could not control her appetite. What she lacked was the critical part of my diet, the mind-body medicines that enable you to control your body, rather than your body controlling you.

I explained my food pyramid to Helen and she left my office vowing to at least give the diet a try. Because she was skeptical, I expected never to see her again; yet, two weeks later she returned, having lost 11 pounds. During the next three months, Helen achieved her goal of losing 40 pounds. She never did lose that healthy skepticism about the diet, despite her success. She was so grateful for the mind-body medicines that she was beside herself. She was able to get through one of the most stressful periods of her life, a divorce, without gaining weight.

## Dr. Fred's Thin For Good Pyramids

Now, I'd like to share my version of the food pyramid with you so that you may better understand how your body metabolizes food, how your new diet works, and what you should be eating. But first, we must review the terribly outdated USDA Daily Food Guide Pyramid. This pyramid is flawed and is giving many people the wrong ideas about what they should be eating. It was especially distressing to me when I learned that this is the one nutritional thing that is stressed in our children's elementary school education. It's no wonder that our kids today have the weight problems they do—they are learning how to eat incorrectly right from the start. Here is this pyramid:

USDA Daily Food Guide Pyramid

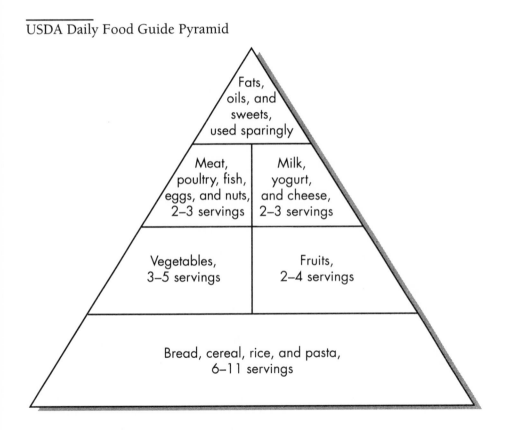

The fatal flaw in this pyramid is its assumption that all grains are created equal. As you will recall from an earlier chapter, insulin and glucose responses to carbohydrate ingestion vary according to the carbohydrate source. As a result, it does matter to your body whether you are getting, for example, white bread or brown rice. Whole grains ought to be differentiated from the simple grains, and adjustments made accordingly.

In Dr. Fred's Thin For Good Pyramid 1 (below), you can see how the body uses what we eat for fuel to produce energy. It is an inverted pyramid that represents the types of food that people will generally eat in a day—the larger the box, the more of it that is eaten.

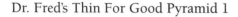

Dr. Fred's Thin For Good Pyramid 1

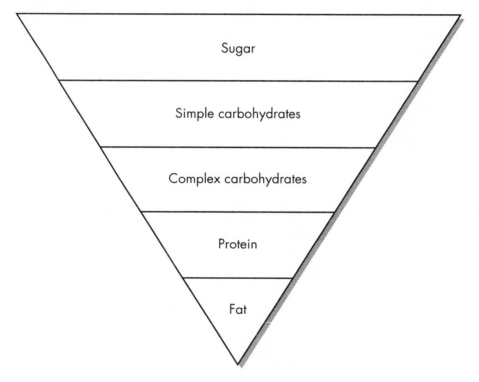

For its energy requirements, the body will start at the top of this pyramid and work its way down. Sugar and simple carbohydrates are less complex molecules and therefore easier for the body to break down. Your body has been doing things this way since the beginning of time.

Your body works its way down this pyramid until it no longer needs any fuel. For example, if there is any sugar present, your body utilizes that for energy. When the sugar is gone, it will use simple carbohydrates. When all of those are used, it will convert complex carbohydrates into energy, then protein, and lastly fat. Everything you eat that the body does not use for energy gets stored, usually in the form of fat.

## The Secrets of Storing Energy

The body works this way because fat is the most efficient storage form of energy. If you eliminate any of the easy-to-digest foods along the top of this pyramid, your body will have to use complex carbohydrates, protein, and fat for its energy needs.

This is precisely how my diet works. By eliminating all the "easy" foods—that is, those that are metabolized first—this diet gets your body to operate at its most efficient level by utilizing the sources of fuel that are the most primitive. That's how you can eat foods that may be high in calories. Keep in mind that prehistoric people had no convenience stores from which to get simple carbohydrates and sugars. They ate only what was caught or picked. It was millions of years before people started to harvest grains and sugars.

## How to Use This Information

You can use my new and improved dietary pyramid to lose weight. Whenever you desire a certain food or are looking for something to eat to stem your hunger, just make sure that the food is part of the bottom two or three categories of Dr. Fred's Thin For Good Pyramid 2 (below). Pyramid 2 shows you how I believe you should be eating foods. The amount of foods you should eat from each category will be based on the stage of the diet you're in. The simple rule to remember is that if the food is in the top two categories of the pyramid, avoid them. It's that easy.

---

Dr. Fred's Thin For Good Pyramid 2

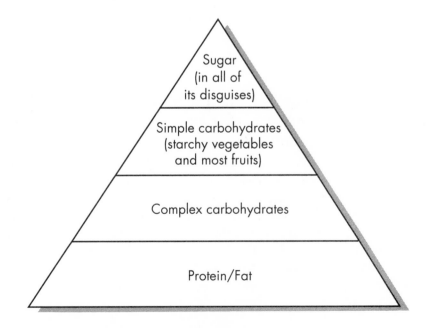

Sugar
(in all of
its disguises)

Simple carbohydrates
(starchy vegetables
and most fruits)

Complex carbohydrates

Protein/Fat

## THE ELEVEN EMOTIONAL LEVELS OF EATING
# LEVEL 4: FEAR

Ironically, fear is an emotion that can be liberating for many of my over-weight patients. Fear often starts to appear after some of the other more obvious emotions have been discussed. It may come up when you are beginning to have a little success with your diet. It may even come up because others are starting to take notice of your success. How does being noticed make you feel? Being successful at a diet? Losing weight? Pretty scary things for someone who has a weight problem.

Fear may be one of the hardest emotions to let go of, especially when you think of dieting in terms of a lifetime. There are two ways look at fear: positive and negative. The negative side of fear is the most obvious, the fear of being thin. After all, when was the last time you were thin? What does being thin really mean to you? These can be extremely real fears for some of us and may be the main obstacle to overcome in your quest for thinness.

On the positive side, I use the fear of ever being overweight again to help ensure that I will always stay within my dietary plan. This can help you as it has helped me. This is a main focus in my mind-body plan—harnessing the tremendous brain power we have and enlisting it to work in our favor, not against us.

Let's explore some of your fears by answering the following questions truthfully:

1. What am I afraid of?
2. Who am I afraid of?
3. What makes me stay awake at night?
4. What worries me?
5. What do I fear the most?


***Bonus Questions: Why do I fear any of these things? Are these fears rational or irrational? Do I have the power to change any of these fears into positives?***

These questions and the answers that go with them may seem completely incompatible to you, but I can assure you they are not. Whether the fear is irrational or not or whether you feel you can change things in order to make them less fearful is irrelevant. What matters most is that you understand your fears are very real and may be the key to what is holding you back from being a successful dieter. Use the mind-body medicines to help you work through these very real fears. If you don't, you will be on the dieting yo-yo your whole life.

**Mind-Body Medicines That May Help Overcome Fear:**
- Stop building walls against losing weight.
- Your desire to be thin can only be achieved through positive behaviors.
- There can be no limitations in your consciousness to get thinner and healthier.

**Recipes That May Help with Fear**
- Cold Sesame Chicken Salad
- Classic Chicken Melt

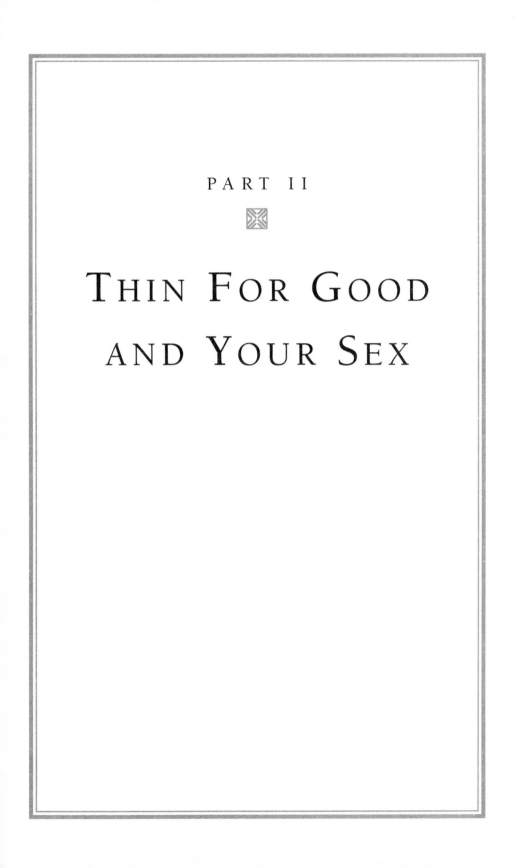

PART II

THIN FOR GOOD
AND YOUR SEX

# ⬚

# CHAPTER 5

# The Gender Gap

Paulette, thirty-six, came to my office because she needed to lose about 15 pounds. It was the first time in her life that she found the previously simple task of dieting quite daunting. Over the past several years she had tried several diet programs, with pretty much the same disastrous results. She would lose one pound the first week, then nothing in subsequent weeks, no matter how strictly she kept to the particular diet.

You might suspect that Paulette wasn't really being truthful with herself while she was on these diets, that perhaps she was not following the rules of the diet to the letter but, as I found out during our conversation, this was simply not the case. Paulette was a career-oriented young woman who led a very structured life and she was driven and determined to achieve no matter what the circumstances were.

The only diet that had achieved any kind of success for her during the past year was a liquid diet drink that by the third week had made her sick to her stomach. It's true she lost 10 pounds in those three weeks, but she quickly gained back those 10 and even added another 5 pounds as soon as she stopped using the drink.

Since Paulette had always been able to lose weight in the past, she became frustrated, and that's when she came to see me, desperate for help. She thought she was doing everything right. She had read everything she could on dieting, and literally had tried every diet, including other low-carbohydrate diets. What intrigued her the most about my diet was what her friend had told her about the mind-body medicines. She was really intrigued by the idea because it made perfect sense to her.

I told Paulette that she fit into the young woman stage of life (see chapter 6 for the description of this type). Then I explained the Mind Over Calories concept to her and provided her with all the mind-body medicines, which she used on her way to the office each morning.

I knew she would do everything perfectly, and she did. She lost 3 pounds the first week, 1 pound the second week, 2 pounds the third week, and managed to drop the 15 pounds she wanted to lose in two and a half months.

Not bad, considering that her weight loss was an impossible feat before she discovered my diet.

Harry, a forty-two-year-old father of two, came to my office because his wife wanted to lose weight and thought it would be a good idea if he did it along with her. Although he had about 20 pounds to lose, Harry didn't consider himself overweight; in fact, he didn't even want to lose weight. He was visiting me under protest and this was made perfectly clear from the outset. He wanted to help his wife, but he was not going to follow any of the advice I might have for him once he was out of his wife's field of vision.

Obviously, this was not a great way to start a new dietary program, but it was not unusual. Like most men, Harry tended to think of himself as being in the same athletic shape and being the same virile man he was in college. But Harry hadn't been to the gym in about four years and any resemblance to the man he was in college was purely coincidental.

When Harry got on the scale in my office and I finally had him alone, away from his wife, I was better able to talk to him about the real issues at hand. The plain fact was that he was 20 pounds overweight. Harry had to look at the scale twice before it sank in that he actually was overweight. He knew his clothes weren't fitting as well as they could have, but 20 pounds? But since most scales don't lie, Harry had to accept this truth. And let's face it, those 20 pounds somehow have a way of creeping up on us, don't they?

I explained to Harry that men and women need different diets in order to be successful. These diets may, in fact, be similar, but with enough differences to make each unique. I also told him that he fit into my weekend warrior stage of life (see chapter 7 for the description of this type). After I explained all the metabolic differences men experience as they age, Harry, always skeptical, leaned back in his chair, looked at me for a minute and said, "I don't think I'm that overweight, and I still don't want to do this, but I'll give it a try for my wife, because she really needs to lose weight. I'm not going to recite those mantras, though."

After two weeks on the diet, Harry had lost 8 pounds. He returned to my office and reported to me that since he was finding the diet so easy to follow, he thought he would continue to give it a try. He even sneaked in one of those silly sayings, as he called them, and admitted it actually helped with a food craving he was having one day. It wasn't long before he found that his clothes were starting to fit better, and so, cheered by these results, he decided to continue on the diet. When I asked him about getting back to exercise, he smiled and said, "Don't press your luck, Doc." I smiled, too, knowing that you can't win all the battles all the time.

Fast forward to one year later: Harry had lost the entire 20 pounds he needed to in less than eight weeks. He found his energy level had improved, as did his sex life. He was so thrilled (and I'm sure his wife was, too) that he eventually even went back to exercising.

Two different people, two different sexes and two similar, but different diets. Both were successful, but neither could have been on the other's diet. Before I explain the way I decide the stages and into which stage a person falls, I would like to discuss the differences between men and women and why these stages are important determinants in how you lose weight.

## The Diet Solution for Women and Men

Because of the differences between men and women, there cannot be a one-diet-fits-all approach to weight loss. I believe that succumbing to this one-diet-fits-all fallacy has gotten many dieters in trouble, because it sets you up to fail. If you can't be as perfect as your husband/boyfriend/wife/lover/neighbor/friend, then you must have been doing something wrong.

How did that make you feel? How does that continue to make you feel? Depressed, miserable, frustrated, exhausted, burnt-out, lonely? Of course it does, but it doesn't have to. Thin For Good will provide the mind-body tools necessary to ensure that, although there are differences in our genetics that determine how we lose or retain weight, we can all get through this. You will be successful because you will learn how to handle the obstacles and pitfalls. We are all individuals and must be treated that way. You can turn all those negative dieting moods into much more positive ones. Wouldn't it be nice to be happy once in a while?

## Women, Men, and Metabolism

Simply put, metabolism is the minimum amount of energy that is required by your body to do its daily tasks, such as breathing and the other bodily functions you take for granted.

Are the metabolisms of men and women different? Absolutely! Men tend to have more muscle mass than women. Women tend to have more fat on their bodies. Because of this, pound for pound, it takes more energy and more calories for the overweight man to maintain his metabolism than it takes for the overweight woman to do the same. Consequently, if you're a woman and you have the same amount of weight to lose as your male counterpart and you eat the very same foods in the very same amounts, he will still lose weight faster, simply because fat takes very little energy to maintain, and biologically a man's body contains more muscle than fat. That's the way it is and there's not much anyone can do about it. What can be done is to make these differences work *for* you, not against you. You need to be on a diet that is best suited for you.

In any weight-loss program there should be an emphasis on exercise so that you can build more muscle. Even at rest, as when you are sleeping, the more muscular, or better-toned, person will burn more calories. This is because muscle tone is necessary even when we sleep, and maintaining this muscle tone burns more calories than maintaining fat.

From the beginning, women are at a definite disadvantage. The metabolic rate of a woman is 10 percent lower than that of a man. For both sexes, this metabolic rate will decrease by 0.5 to 1 percent each year, starting at about age twenty-five. This decrease essentially goes unnoticed until the age of about thirty-five to forty, when suddenly you get on the scale, and realize, "Oh, no, I've gained 10 pounds."

Men don't have all the advantages, because women are much better dieters than men. That is mostly because women tend to be more cerebral when it comes to dieting. They have the psychological edge. The women in my practice almost always use the mind-body tools, whereas the men use them about 65 percent of the time. *By using the mind-body tools and the diet that is specific to sex and stage of life, I have been able to eliminate the physical advantage men have over women.* By the same token, I have been able to increase men's staying power on the diet by giving them a diet they can live with over the long haul.

Women are better able to maximize their choices within a narrow range of food groups to keep their life, and their diet, interesting. They therefore tend to get less bored with their diet and are motivated to continue. Women are also usually better able to take care of themselves and the men in their lives from a medical standpoint. They are more comfortable spending time on themselves, and this often crosses over to their health.

Men are more likely than women to resist seeing themselves as overweight. Because of this, they are also more likely to put off doing anything about the problem until they or someone they know has suffered from some of the negative consequences associated with obesity, namely heart disease or diabetes. My diet is perfect for men because it addresses their most common health concerns.

Women tend to have an easier time at dieting for another reason. I'm sure that has something to say about our society. Keep in mind that self-esteem for women peaks at age nine, whereas men's self-esteem increases as they age. Women are supposed to be thin and great-looking and have fabulous careers and families in order to be deemed successful. Men often only need to have a good career to be deemed successful.

I want you to be able to learn to use the psychic energy of dieting for good causes and not negative ones. Usually, the desires and cravings that we experience often overwhelm us and cause us to go off a diet. Mind Over Calories will help you channel these urges so you stay on the program rather than fall off. *You are going to learn that this psychic energy that you consider negative can really be put to positive uses.* Mind Over Calories is something even men can do.

## Men and the Mind-Body Medicines

Men like to get results, and the quicker the better. Generally, men are more result-oriented than women and are often unwilling to wait long for those results to occur. Amazingly, I have had male patients complain that their weight loss was not quick enough, despite their averaging 4 to 6 pounds per week.

Because of their need for quick results, men usually don't learn how to lose weight. This is where the Mind Over Calories concept comes in quite handy. It has been an invaluable tool in both my own and my patients' ability to lose weight and successfully keep it off. The device works well for women who are more comfortable exploring alternative avenues in the quest for thinness and in men who need to learn how to use the power of their minds for something other than success on the ball field or at their jobs.

## Women and Men and Cravings

Clara, a thirty-nine-year-old unmarried woman, came to my office for a follow-up visit. She was very upset because she had fallen off her diet. She was having a particularly troubling time recently, because she had broken up with her boyfriend and, as a result, needed to find a new apartment. Anyone familiar with the real estate market in New York City can appreciate how troublesome and anxiety provoking that scenario can be, let alone having to deal with the emotions of breaking up with one's significant other.

In this time of trouble, who do you think Clara turned to? Her good friend, chocolate.

In my practice, the association between women and chocolate seems to be one of life's givens. Recently, modern science has caught up to this observation and has begun to investigate why women seem to love, even crave chocolate. In most scientific studies, women rate sweets as their number one food craving. It shouldn't come as a surprise that this craving is so intense, because several studies have shown a biological basis for the need for something sweet.

Men also have crutches. This crutch usually takes the form of alcohol, but may be something salty, like potato chips.

I once appeared on a television show on Valentine's Day to discuss the subject of women and chocolate. I was reporting on a study that demonstrated that the substance in chocolate that women were really craving was phenylethalamine, or PEA. This substance acts as a brain neurotransmitter to make an individual feel less depressed, and it functions somewhat like Prozac by mimicking your brain chemistry. In times of stress or during periods of sadness, it was found that women craved something to alleviate that depression and that it was the PEA in chocolate that they craved.

The latest study conducted on this subject shows that not all women are so chocolate obsessed. Spanish women who crave sweets, for example, are considerably less attached to chocolate, and are no more enamored of it than Spanish men are. This revelation causes us to take another look at the chocolate phenomenon. As a result, it's now believed that perhaps the reason American women crave chocolate more than women in other cultures is that people tend to crave and enjoy familiar foods when they're under emotional stress. And chocolate is very familiar.

## Examine Your Motives

The truth is, we *learn* our addictions and our cravings. When we reach for food in troubled times, we almost always go back to the foods that made us feel good as children, foods our mothers fed us.

If this is true, then it must be possible to retrain ourselves to desire different foods when we experience these troubling periods—foods that are actually healthy. *The way we eat is nothing more than a series of habits. We just need to learn better habits.*

When I introduce my diet to new people, they often say in so many words that there is no way they will ever be able to stay on the diet, yet most of them are remarkably successful once they've allowed themselves to relearn their eating rituals. We must constantly strive to learn new eating habits. I don't think there's a reader of this book who can truthfully say that his or her eating habits are good, let alone perfect.

You need to examine your motives when it comes to food. You must answer the question What does food mean to me? Is it comfort? Is it pleasure? Or is it just sustenance? The answer to these questions is of the utmost importance and, ultimately, the key to understanding why you eat the way you do. It is the only way you will finally be able to break the cycle of poor eating habits and yo-yo dieting.

The Thin For Good program has eliminated many of the discrepancies between the sexes, so that it is easy for men and women to lose weight together and to keep it off for the rest of their lives without killing each other in the process.

## The Sexes—Advantages vs. Disadvantages

### Advantages

*Male*

Higher metabolic rate

More muscle mass, less fat

Easier to lose weight

Better self-esteem

*Female*

Better dieters

Maximizers of food choices

Better motivation

Use mind-body medicines
close to 100%

Take better care of
themselves

### Disadvantages

*Male*

Worse dieters

Less motivated to lose weight

Make poor food choices

Resist seeing themselves as
overweight

Not used to suffering for vanity

Take less care of themselves

Use mind-body medicines 65%

*Female*

Lower metabolic rate

Less muscle mass, more
body fat

Harder to lose weight

Less self-esteem

# THE ELEVEN EMOTIONAL LEVELS OF EATING
## LEVEL 5: UNDERSTANDING

At last we come to some of the more positive emotions. It has been my experience that most of us go through more negative than positive emotions when it comes to dieting. After we get through blame and guilt and everything that has come before, we are finally ready to understand what is going on in our minds when it comes to dieting and our desire to be healthier and thinner. By this point, we have begun to understand some of the forces that have made us gain weight, and we will be able to use this new knowledge to forge ahead and make some real, positive improvements.

At this point, we need to have a more healthy understanding of the pitfalls that will accompany us along the road to wellness. We must also acknowledge that although we may understand that there are many negative obstacles, this understanding alone doesn't make it any easier.

Knowing that the obstacles are there, and knowing that something is going to be difficult, helps us do the right thing. All too often, patients think that now that they have found the diet that is right for them, all will be well, their lives will be easier, their problems solved. This is true only if you acknowledge that you must do some mind-body work along the way. The real understanding comes when you understand the real reason you are overweight or unhealthy.

Explore these questions to help you figure out this concept:

1. What have I come to understand about myself?
2. What do I understand about my eating habits?
3. What do I understand about the people in my life and their effect on my dieting?
4. What pitfalls are going to make this road harder?
5. What do I appreciate most about what I have learned?

## Bonus Question: Does having a real understanding make anything easier for me?

This is the hardest thing to answer about this emotion. What does understanding really mean? What effects will it have on your life? Understanding everything you may be going through emotionally when it comes to dieting is essential to moving through the levels. However, it is not the last level, by a long shot.

### Mind-Body Medicines for Understanding

- You must have more than a momentary commitment to being thinner.

- What do I need to learn from being overweight?
- What am I supposed to learn from this bagel?

**Recipes That May Help with Understanding**
- Classic Salmon
- V's Arrosto Di Vitello

# CHAPTER 6

# The Female Diet Stages

Research has shown that men and women respond differently to everything from pain medication to heart attacks, and now new FDA regulations ensure the inclusion of women in most major relevant clinical trials. Recently it has been shown that female athletes perform better when their diets are higher in fat. These women are urged to focus less on carbohydrates and more on fat.

There is a whole new world out there in terms of women's health, and this must be taken into consideration when selecting a dietary program for yourself and your loved ones.

## Estrogen and Weight Control

Do you crave sugar and other sweet foods more when you are premenstrual than at any other time of the month? You probably do, because there is a metabolic process that occurs between estrogen, which decreases in the days before the menstrual cycle, and the rest of your body's hormones, especially insulin. Estrogen tends to regulate a woman's secretion of insulin, helping keep that all-important balance. Estrogen in a woman's bloodstream will keep insulin levels lower than they would otherwise be.

Without the regulating effect of estrogen, the secretion of insulin will continue to increase when you eat, without any stabilizer. This matters because insulin is a storage hormone that tells your body to pack away any calories that may be around. High insulin levels lead to high amounts of storage. Tell me you've never felt as if your body just didn't want to get rid of anything at that time of the month.

Insulin will also cause your blood sugar to fall. That is what it is supposed to do. However, too much insulin will cause your blood sugar to drop too much, leading to sugar cravings, hunger pangs, and even—in extreme cases—passing out. Because you have a craving for sugar and there is still too much insulin around, the excess sugar that is floating around your bloodstream will be stored as excess fat. So, you can see that food cravings and mood swings have a physiological basis during your menstrual cycle.

I have many satisfied female patients simply because I recognize the need to put women on a diet that is specifically suited for them. Women need to regulate their blood sugar even more than men because women tend to get more symptomatic. They will feel it more. My diet will solve this problem before your next menstrual cycle if you follow the rules. But first, you have to determine which stage of life you are in.

## The Female Stages

You already know that I believe men and women should be on different diets, but I also feel that there are certain identifiable variables for each sex when it comes to losing weight. In my years of experience with the many women I have treated, I have seen a general pattern emerge that corresponds to certain stages of life. These stages usually have to do with age, but not always.

To better help me illustrate the various stages, I am going to give you a case history for each that will help you determine into which stage you may fall, as there is a different diet for each female stage. Don't worry if none of the characteristics of these women seem to correspond to you, or if you find that you are a little bit of each stage. At the end of this chapter you'll find a quiz to help you determine your stage and which diet you should follow.

### The Beginners

Jane, twenty-five, came into my office simply to lose 10 pounds and to get on a program that she could live with for the rest of her life. She was having some difficulty keeping excess weight off, despite the fact that she exercised four nights a week. She was also unsure as to how she was ever going to stay on any sort of diet program because she ate dinner out most nights of the week as well as lunch every day. She did not have the time to cook at home, and since her mother never cooked either, she barely knew how to boil water. She needed an easy-to-follow, step-by-step program that she didn't have to think about too much. She also knew that if a diet or nutritional program was ever going to work, she needed to be realistic and she needed to have, as she put it, her "head wrapped around it." She had never had a weight problem before and attributed the one she had now to going out with friends after work most nights for dinner and drinks. She was young, single, and out to have a good time. How, she wondered, was she ever going to fit dieting into this schedule?

I assured Jane that my program would provide her with a diet that was specific for her stage in life, and would give her the psychological tools nec-

essary to get her head wrapped around it, and to make a lifestyle change—
the key to any successful diet. Jane especially loved the quiz I had her take
before she could get on my program. Like many of us, she loved taking
quizzes in all the health magazines she devoured at the gym.

The beginner woman is generally between the ages of eighteen and
thirty-two, bent on making a name for herself in the world. She is usually
single, supporting herself, and often lives on her own. She is an avid exer-
ciser and keeps up-to-date on women's issues through all the magazines she
reads. She is biologically more likely to begin a family, and can generally lose
weight fairly easily.

In fact, women in the beginner stage lose weight much as men do, especially if they are physically active. These women tend to be mesomorphic in
their body type—athletic and muscular. Although for many women it may
be easy to lose weight in this stage, for others it may not, because a woman's
genetic imprinting predisposes her to begin retaining body fat for the potential growth of a fetus during pregnancy. There may be other factors as well
that will prevent some women in this category from losing weight, such
as thyroid disease, or other inheritable character traits, such as obesity or
diabetes in the family.

### Young Women

Paula, thirty-nine, had just had her first baby three weeks before seeing me.
She wanted to start on a good nutritional program to lose the weight of
pregnancy before she got back to work in the next five weeks. She also
wanted time to practice and get everything just right before starting full
speed at her job.

Paula had gained 55 pounds during her pregnancy because she ate whatever she wanted to. It was the first time in her life that she had allowed herself such an indulgence, and she was finding it difficult to get back on the
right track. She still exercised twice a week, but was concerned that with a
new baby she would never be able to maintain the workout schedule she
thought was the key to keeping her weight down. This was the first time in
her life she had been overweight and she did not like the way it felt. She was
ready to dedicate herself to a new lifestyle change, whatever it took. Paula
approached most things this way, and this was the main reason she was successful, both professionally and personally. It was now up to me to get her
into the shape she wanted to be. She gave me two weeks to see results before
she was off to the next doctor.

Generally, the young woman aged thirty-three to forty-three finds that
for the first time in her life weight loss doesn't come so easily, even if it
always did in the past. The amount of exercise, the amount of food, and the
lifestyle may not have changed at all, and yet the weight just doesn't seem

to come off. In fact, she gains weight each year, much more easily than ever before. This is especially the case today, when many women in this age bracket first begin families. The weight will go on during pregnancy and it doesn't seem to want to go away as readily as it once did. The main reason the new extra pounds are difficult to shed could be slowing of the metabolism—a serious, often derided, but all-too-true reason for weight gain at this stage. In this stage most women move from the mesomorphic body type to the endomorphic type.

## Perimenopausal/Menopausal Women

Jackie, fifty, was in the throes of menopause, with hot flashes occurring almost every half hour. She had gained about 25 pounds in the past two years, and was now close to 50 pounds overweight. She was quite concerned about several issues: the hot flashes, osteoporosis, and weight gain. She attributed the weight gain to the change of life she was experiencing, as all her friends had had the same thing happen to them. Little did she know that the weight gain did not have to happen. All Jackie needed was a diet specific to her stage in life.

I don't think there is another diet book that offers the reader a diet specific for the perimenopausal/menopausal female. The needs are very specific and different and must be taken into consideration if you are ever to expect to lose weight at this point in your life.

Jackie did not have a career. She stayed at home, and now that her kids were gone, she found herself eating a little too much, going out to lunch with her friends a little too often, and busying herself with so many little things that she wasn't even playing tennis as often as she once did. She was especially concerned after reading that overweight women have an increased risk of getting breast cancer because excess estrogen is stored in the fatty tissues, which may lead to breast cancer. Jackie had tried so many diets, including all the popular low-carbohydrate diets, and naturally she was wondering what was different about my diet.

I had to convince her to give it a try by telling her that my diet not only has a specific plan for her stage in life, but that it holds the key to successful weight loss—a mind-body program designed specifically to help her break through the plateaus that are so easily reached in a perimenopausal/menopausal woman. This mind-body program would not fail her in her quest to lose weight.

The perimenopausal/menopausal woman is forty-four to fifty-five years old and generally has the most difficulty losing weight. However, since the metabolic changes associated with menopause may start much earlier than this, the quiz at the end of this chapter may place you in this category even if your age is not in this range. If you are in this group, your menstrual cycle may or may not still be regular and you may or may not have hot flashes or any of the other overt signs that you've always associated with menopause. But there may be other subtle symptoms, such as a memory that is not as razor sharp as it once was, thinning hair and less strong nails, even a lessening of the libido. These bodily changes can and often do affect weight loss in a negative way.

## Postmenopausal Women

Cynthia, sixty-two, came to see me because she had gained 35 pounds during menopause and had virtually given up trying to lose weight until she felt she was through with those changes. Over the years, she had tried many diets: low-fat, low-carbohydrate, liquid fasts—all with the same negative results. So inevitably she gave up! Not that anyone could blame her. She was on the one-diet-fits-all approach that simply didn't take into account that people need to be on different diets as they age and as they approach different stages of their lives. Cynthia was finally disgusted enough with herself that she thought she would give my diet a try, as I had been able to help several of her friends who were in the same boat.

Cynthia, a grandmother whose daughter was busy with her career, really dedicated her life to taking care of her grandchildren. She was especially motivated to lose weight because she was having increasing difficulty keeping up with their active lives. Summer was coming and she didn't want to be the fattest grandmother at the swim club, so this was also a big inspiration to her. Cynthia was very content with her life. She had retired from her activities at the local hospital, where she had been a director of human resources, and wanted to spend the next couple of years (before her husband retired and they moved south) enjoying her grandkids, especially before they grew too old to appreciate her. Her only real problem was that she was just very disappointed and frustrated with her weight. She was reluctant to try yet another diet and spend more money on something that may not be successful. If it weren't for her friends doing so well on my diet, she would not have been in my office.

Cynthia wanted a program that could help her through the hard times and give her some emotional support along the way. Little did she know that losing weight at this stage in her life was going to be easier than at any time since her mid-forties.

The postmenopausal woman is generally above the age of fifty-six and is finally finished with the symptoms of menopause. She is the woman many younger women aspire to be—she has all the knowledge and can pass it on to her younger cohorts. Some call this period of life the golden years. Life tends to get easier. Most working women are retired at this point or are looking forward to retirement and the lessening of responsibilities that comes along with that. The mortgage is paid, the children are raised, and after enjoying the grandchildren all day, she can go home and enjoy the peace and quiet. A woman is even said to look her best at this time in her life, and I think that comes from the inner sense of serenity that she must feel, knowing that life is now hers to enjoy without all the battles. It is even easier to lose weight in this stage than in some of the younger ones.

Women in this stage begin to require more nutritional supplements than ever before. This is partly due to the aging process; the body has a decreased ability to absorb nutrients from the foods we eat. But also, as we age, our requirements increase to help fight the battles of aging. So, even if you have never taken nutritional supplements in the past, now is the time to begin.

Needless to say, all four of these women found that being on a diet that was specifically geared for their stage of life enabled them to lose weight, and as a result, they were very pleased. Their energy levels improved and so did their outlook on life. They were suddenly feeling less depressed. They also found the mind-body medicines to be an extremely helpful tool that really helped get their psyches aligned with their bodies. When trying to lose weight, this is something that can't be ignored. Focus and concentration usually make the difference.

## Figuring Out Your Stage

It is possible that the four women I have just described bear little resemblance to you. This doesn't mean, however, that we won't be able to figure out your stage of life. *The stages are not just age related.* That is why it is necessary to take the following quiz.

This quiz is going to be evaluated on a point system, and the number of points you have at the end of the quiz will determine your stage of life and where to begin Thin For Good's initiation phase. Please be honest, because if you aren't you will only hurt yourself and possibly jeopardize your chances to lose weight by not allowing yourself to be placed in the category in which you really belong. Please don't be upset by the category into which you may fall. A twenty-two-year-old may fall into the perimenopausal/menopausal category and a sixty-year-old may, too. It doesn't matter. What matters is that you find your stage, have a successful outcome, and have fun along the way.

1. Are you between the ages of 18 and 32? (3 points)
2. Are you between the ages of 33 and 43? (6 points)
3. Are you between the ages of 44 and 55? (9 points)
4. Are you above the age of 56? (12 points)
5. Do you exercise less than 3 times per week? (2 points)

6. Do you exercise more than 5 times per week?     (minus 1 point)

7. Have you ever had a baby?     (1 point)

8. Do you have a history of an underactive thyroid?     (2 points)

9. Does obesity run in your family?     (1 point)

10. Does diabetes run in your family?     (1 point)

11. Are your menstrual periods regular?     (Yes = minus 1 point; No = 1 point)

12. Do you have a decreased sex drive?     (1 point)

13. Is it easy for you to lose weight?     (minus 1 point)

14. Is it easy for you to follow the rules of a diet perfectly?  (minus 1 point)

15. Is your favorite food from the sugar family?     (2 points)

If your total is:

- 1 to 5 points:  This makes you a beginner. Begin with that section of the initiation phase specifically for your stage and don't forget to use the mind-body medicines.

- 6 to 9 points:  This makes you the young woman. You are going to have a great time on the diet. Please go to the section of the initiation phase that pertains to your stage.

- 10 to 16 points:  This makes you the perimenopausal/menopausal female. Good luck with your new lifestyle regimen. You are going to love a diet that is made specifically for you.

- 17 points and above:  This places you in the postmenopausal category. Congratulations and please refer to the diet that is made especially for you.

## Where to Go from Here

Your next step, no matter what stage you fall into, is to read chapter 8 on the initiation phase for all stages, which I like to call the guiding principles. Don't forget to read the Eleven Emotional Levels of Eating at the end of each chapter, even if the chapter doesn't apply to you. Chapter 8 will provide you with the basic rules that anyone on this diet must follow. Although there are specific stages and certain restrictions for each stage, these diets are not so radically different from each other that you will not be able to diet with your friends or family if you decide to do this together and they fall into a different stage. Once you've mastered the guiding principles, move on to chapter 9 for the diets for the different female stages and follow your individual stage. Good luck—and most important—have fun.

# THE ELEVEN EMOTIONAL LEVELS OF EATING
## LEVEL 6: TREPIDATION

Nervousness, edginess, wariness. This level of emotion goes by many names, but it all boils down to the same thing: fear of the unknown. Most people get to this level roughly halfway or three quarters of the way through the initiation phase of their diet. They can see their thinner selves, feel the success, know that it is just around the corner, and then the doubt begins to set in. What life is going to be like as a thin person is what they are most afraid of.

This is a completely natural phenomenon. Most people will have an understanding of some of their emotions and feelings by this point as they relate to dieting, but now the true edge is there. It is real and can cut like a knife. This is the stage where many people truly will break their diet, if only momentarily. This momentary lapse can have long-term implications in their struggle with weight, because it can undermine everything that has come before. This is different from fear, because at the fear point, the dieter is generally afraid of everything—not knowing what is going to happen, not knowing if the diet is even going to be successful.

At this point, you know the success you will be having and how good you will feel. The question is: Can you tolerate feeling good? I know this may sound strange, but it is an emotion that many of my patients have experienced. Can you continue with this? Is sugar something you are willing to mostly give up for the rest of your life? These are serious questions, and this is the stage where those doubts seriously can impede your progress if you are not aware that they exist and—most important—that they can be overcome.

You are about to jump off the cliff—do you dare?

Here are some questions that may help you realize how easily this feeling of trepidation can be overcome, and that you can be a successful dieter for life:

1. What makes me nervous about food?
2. What foods do I think I can't live without?
3. Who makes me nervous?
4. What makes me nervous in general?
5. When in my life do I experience the most trepidation?

### Bonus Question: Can I live with a certain level of trepidation in my life?

This is truly the key to getting through this phase. I think the answer is yes, because so often we live with fear on an almost daily basis, and do perfectly well. And I don't mean fear for our safety. Many of us are afraid of something to do with our careers. Many of us feel trepidation about an exam, a new assignment, raising the children properly, whatever. However, we always manage to get through those fears because we have to in order to survive and be successful. Why should it be any different when it comes to food? The standards we set for our dieting lives have to be just as high as those we set for the rest of our lives.

### Mind-Body Medicines for Trepidation
- Energy has no limitations in our drive for thinness.
- There can be no limitations in our consciousness to get thinner and healthier.
- You are in this dieting game—play it for all it's worth.

### Recipes That May Help with Trepidation
- Tropical Cucumbers
- Greek Quinoa

# CHAPTER 7

# The Male Diet Stages

Matt, forty-four, came into my office one day and I asked him, as I generally ask all my patients, "What brings you here today?" The answer I usually look for is the person's chief complaint. What I'm really asking is, "What's wrong with you? What made you want to see a doctor?" The answer I got from Matt was one that was not unfamiliar to me: "I'm here because my wife wanted me to come." Matt was deadly serious. He felt there was no reason at all to be in my office. He felt great, had loads of energy, and couldn't understand why his wife was putting him through such torture.

After reviewing all of Matt's blood work, I could see several areas that needed work, primarily his cholesterol. Matt's cholesterol was 275, with an HDL (the good cholesterol) of 35. His triglycerides were 312. These numbers were terrible, and they put Matt at the highest risk for heart disease. As it happened, Matt's father and grandfather both had had heart attacks at age fifty and, from the looks of these numbers, Matt was on the same track. And to make matters worse, he was 40 pounds overweight.

Matt really felt he had no problem. After all, he had not changed any of his habits since college, and if they worked for him then, why wouldn't they work for him now?

He hadn't the first clue about the state of his health, and he had no interest in finding out. Despite all his protests, I gave Matt such an easy diet for him to follow, one that suited him so perfectly, that I knew he would be able to do this with ease. Within two weeks, Matt had lost 11 pounds by making a few adjustments to his eating habits, and by reading and studying a few mind-body medicines.

Matt is not unlike most men in that we tend to take diets and dieting for granted. We just eat without considering the consequences, because, generally speaking, we can, thanks to our metabolism. As a rule, most men tend to eat larger quantities of food than women. There is a certain inherent male quality that makes men want to "pack it away," almost as if it's a badge of honor.

For my male patients, this particular eating habit is the one that is incredibly difficult to break. It is a habit men learn from a very early age. It is even part of some of the bonding rituals that men go through—think back to college and those enormous kegs of beer, or the eating contests. Men hardly ever consider the consequences of getting older and therefore don't feel the need to change the way they eat as they age. However, as we get older, changes must be made in order to satisfy the body's decreasing requirement for energy and the requirement for less food.

## Metabolism and Men

As most men age, owing to the decreased amount of testoterone, they begin to lose muscle mass and their resting metabolic rate decreases, so they will gain weight even without changing their eating habits. Because you will burn less energy while at rest, you will gain two or three pounds for every year over age thirty if you don't change your eating habits. No one is immune to this phenomenon, unless he is an athlete. Even then, in the off season, he will still have to watch what he eats more closely. This is why so many athletes come to training camp heavier than they were at the end of the previous season. It is a simple rule of biology, and the only way to avoid it is to maintain a proper exercise regime or to control what you eat.

Between the ages of forty and fifty—which I believe is the prime time in a man's life when he will be overweight—men begin to gain weight around the middle. This "middle-age spread" begins gradually. The meso-morphic ideal body type begins to change into the endomorph. Yet in most cases, men are not even aware of this.

The reduction in testosterone that comes as men age can cause many other symptoms, like anxiety and sexual dissatisfaction, a syndrome commonly described as *male menopause*. Men who are more fit than their peers report these symptoms less than their not-so-fit counterparts. Wouldn't you want to do something that would keep your sex drive at its best? This simple diet will enable you to continue to function at your optimum for longer than it would have been possible before—by decreasing the effects of aging.

There are important health benefits to losing weight as a man ages. That is why I have developed certain male stages that will provide men with the diet that is best suited for them. My diet will help you get through some of the more difficult times on this battlefield by providing you with a comprehensive mind-body approach and a diet that is specifically designed for your stage of life.

This book provides you with the answer to why different things happen to you as you enter different stages in your life. It tells you what makes you unique and how you can use that uniqueness to your advantage rather than your disadvantage. Men need to take responsibility for their dieting and other health habits. This plan makes it easy to do that.

It is possible to lose weight and get healthy no matter what type of man you are. For men, the real issue is usually about getting healthy. I believe that if men were just aware of the physiological changes that occur in their bodies, they would be better able to make the necessary adjustments to their diet without the added frustration of thinking they are doing something incorrectly. Let's abandon the frustration; the mind-body exercises will help you to do just that.

## The Different Male Stages

There are fewer male stages than female ones. And in order to make them clearer, I'm going to give you a patient story that describes each stage. Don't be alarmed if these patients do not sound like you. They are only generalizations. So, for the moment, just read along and see if any of the characteristics describe you, as I'm sure they will. At the end of this chapter, you will find a quiz to aid you in determining at which stage you should start.

### The Beginners

Jeff, a thirty-one-year-old police officer, came to my office because he wanted to lose 25 pounds. He had started to gain this weight over the past three years because he had gone from being a beat cop to a detective and he wasn't out on the street chasing criminals as he had been doing for ten years prior to our meeting. He was beginning to see physical changes that he wasn't happy with.

Jeff was an ex-athlete. He had been on all the sports teams in high school, and as a beat cop, exercised religiously four days a week at the gym in the precinct house. He had not changed his eating habits since high school, and he attributed this weight gain to being behind a desk more than ever before in the past. He was definitely becoming more of an endomorph.

Health issues aside, Jeff was unhappy with the way he looked. He was going to be married in four months and wanted to look his best. He wanted a diet that would allow him to lose weight quickly and easily, as well as one that wouldn't make him feel like a rabbit. His fiancée was on a low-calorie diet for the wedding and he knew that there was no way he could be on the same diet she was on. He had tried it, but was too hungry all the time.

Beginners are generally between the ages of eighteen and forty and have never had to diet in their lives. This is the time in men's lives when they are said to be in their prime, when men are most driven to achieve. As men move toward the older end of this spectrum, they begin to realize that they are not indestructible, and that what they did to their bodies as younger men may be having a real impact on their health. I'm often reminded of the comment made about his health by Mickey Mantle, whose father died young: "If I'd have known I was going to live this long, I would have taken better care of myself."

## The Weekend Warriors

Chuck, forty-seven, came to see me for two reasons. The first was obvious. He was 50 pounds overweight and he was no longer able to keep up competitively with his younger racquetball partners. The second reason was that he had had a cholesterol screening at his office and found out that his number was really high and he did not want to take any medication to lower it. He was afraid of the side effects, he said, but it was clear to me that he was really afraid of admitting that he had a health problem.

Chuck was an investment banker. With the economy so strong, he was doing extremely well financially and working very long hours. There was no more time for the gym. When he did have time, his wife and children needed him, so exercising was put on the back burner and there it had stayed for the past three years. The only sport he did play was racquetball once a week, because some of his clients did and it was another opportunity to close a deal. Instead of continuing with and expanding his exercise program, he started to acquire the toys of his generation. He bought a Harley. He went out to eat every night of the week, usually with clients. He traveled around the globe to close deals, ate and drank on airplanes, didn't exercise at the hotel gyms, and made other life choices that soon became part of an unhealthy daily routine. He needed a change and he needed one fast. He was a heart attack waiting to happen.

Chuck needed a diet that would conform to his lifestyle. There was no way I could put him on a diet that required him to cook at home, or that required him to look foolish when he was dining out with clients. He needed a diet that would allow him to be on a diet without looking like he was. I had to explain that although this diet enabled him to do all of those things, he would still have to make a commitment to changing certain things about the way he ate. We don't get overweight without a reason. The weight will not come off and stay off without making some changes. I informed him that it would take two weeks for him to be able to make the necessary adjustments, not only to different foods, but to taking the time to do the mind-body medicines. He reluctantly agreed.

Chuck was a weekend warrior. These men are generally between the ages of forty-one and sixty, when men's driving hormone, testosterone, begins to decline at the rate of approximately 1 percent per year. This is the primary reason why muscle mass in men begins to decline during this period and why men, usually for the first time, find it increasingly difficult to lose weight. If they do manage to lose weight, they have trouble keeping it off. Men will lose 3 to 5 percent of their muscle mass for every decade after age twenty-five. This loss of muscle, coupled with the decrease in physical activity that most men of this age group experience, leads to a decrease in a man's resting metabolic rate.

Since there is often no time for physical activity during the week because of work commitments, exercise becomes relegated to the weekends. Weekend physical activity tends to be more socially driven than physically driven, and the body suffers because of this. Injuries are more common. Injuries prevent you from exercising and then you fall out of the routine and a vicious cycle starts from which you tend not to recover. But you can!

Because of this decline in activity, coupled with the decrease in the testosterone levels, the metabolic advantage that men have previously had over women begins to disappear.

Another problem that arises in men at this stage is the typical weight gain around the middle, which is where most men tend to gain weight as they age. This is especially ominous, because it signifies an insulin resistance problem that can lead to heart disease, high cholesterol, and diabetes. My diet controls blood sugar while helping you lose weight, which is the perfect antidote to that middle age spread and the endomorphic condition.

## The Experienced

Seth, sixty-eight, came to my office because he was concerned about his health. He wanted to lose weight because over the years he had gained about 30 pounds, but he wanted a diet that would keep him healthy so that he could live to see at least 100. He was very active, still working from home as a consultant, but primarily he wanted to live to enjoy his retirement years, and he knew that would be impossible if he continued along the path he was taking. Recently, he had noticed the weight gain and the accompanying shortness of breath. He was at the stage in life when many of his friends were dying—three from heart attacks, four from various cancers—and he was beginning to get worried.

His wife was a patient of mine and he knew how well she was doing since starting the program. She had lost 20 pounds and had more energy than ever before. He wanted that for himself so he could keep up with her. He also wanted to know which supplements he should be taking to protect his heart and prostate.

Experience is the stage of life that usually begins above the age of sixty. The man is retired or thinking about retirement. He is also interested in seeing if anything can be done to keep himself healthy or to get off any medication he may be taking, whether it be for heart trouble, diabetes, prostate, or whatever. He wants to be prepared for the next stage in his life. He has been productive his whole life, and wants to continue to be so through the next few decades. He wants nothing to stop him from enjoying the life he worked so hard to achieve.

In this stage, however, there are certain important things a man needs to consider in his quest for good health. For example, testosterone may begin to exert harmful effects. It can aggravate hair loss; it is the leading cause of baldness in men. But, most important, testosterone can stimulate growth of the prostate gland. Eighty percent of all prostate cancer cases occur in men in this stage.

A man in this stage will continue to lose muscle mass and will continue to put on weight as he ages. Because of this, he will need to ingest fewer calories. Appetites will diminish, but nutritional requirements will increase. This occurs because a man's body may lose its ability to synthesize and absorb vitamins and minerals. This is an essential time in a man's life for him to take nutritional supplements, even if he never has done so in the past.

Not only did each of the men I've just described lose weight on my program, but they also actually enjoyed their diets. They got relatively quick results and were excited to be able to have a diet that was best suited for men and for their particular stage of life. All of them expressed to me how happy they were because they each felt that I had understood them. They weren't just a number, or the next overweight person. They were able to lose weight quickly and easily while getting more energy and feeling better along the way. As an extra bonus, they enjoyed the mind-body part of the diet as well. They never realized how important it was to have their heads in the same place as their bodies. It was almost as if they were thinking themselves thin. They all knew the results they could get when they applied their minds to their careers or their games, but they didn't realize they could focus that energy on losing weight and be successful at the task.

## Determining Your Stage

Here's a simple quiz that will help you determine which stage you belong to. *Remember, it is not strictly determined by age.* Although I have provided age generalities, it is still possible for a young man to be in an older stage and vice versa. It all depends on the outcome of this quiz. Answer all the questions truthfully. You will harm no one other than yourself by trying to fit into a stage that is not right for you.

1. Are you between the ages of 18 and 40?                    (4 points)
2. Are you between the ages of 41 and 60?                    (8 points)
3. Are you older than 60?                                   (12 points)

4. Do you exercise four or more times per week? (minus 2 points)

5. Do you consider yourself a weekend warrior? (minus 1 point)

6. Has your energy level decreased? (1 point)

7. Has your libido decreased? (2 points)

8. Is there a history of diabetes in your family? (1 point)

9. Is there a history of heart disease in your family? (1 point)

10. Do you weigh the same or less than when you graduated from high school? (minus 2 points)

11. Do you weigh the same or less than when you graduated from college? (minus 1 point)

12. Do you smoke? (1 point)

13. Do you have elevated cholesterol? (1 point)

14. Do you tend to gain weight around the middle? (1.5 points)

15. Is this the first time you have ever been overweight in your life? (minus 1 point)

If your total is:

- 0 to 6 points:  You are a beginner. You should follow the instructions that pertain to that stage in the diet for men chapter (chapter 10).

- 7 to 11 points:  This makes you a weekend warrior. Read the guiding principle chapter (chapter 8) first, then go to the specific stage of the initiation phase. Don't forget the mind-body medicines.

- 12 points and above:  This makes you Mr. Experienced. Follow that specific phase of the diet.

## Where to Go From Here

Now that you have figured out the stage of life you are in, the next thing to do is to read chapter 8 on the guiding principles of my diet. This will give you all the basic information you need to know in order to do well, lose weight, and start to feel better. Once you've read the guiding principles, then turn to chapter 10 and find your specific stage (but don't forget to read the Emotional Level of Eating for each chapter) and read about the tactics that will make your diet work the best it can for you. Although the stages are different, they are not so different that you would be unable to diet with a friend, co-worker, or other partner. There are many similarities, so I encourage you to do this with a partner if you can.

So read on. Don't forget the mind-body medicines, as they play a key role. And have fun along the way.

## THE ELEVEN EMOTIONAL LEVELS OF EATING
# LEVEL 7: ENVY

Once you have come to this stage, you may be envious of those around you. After all, how many times in the past have you tried to diet and had someone do better than you, lose weight faster than you, lose more weight than you did? Or worse yet, have an easier time at it than you? I have to admit that I have always been envious of those who didn't want to lose weight or didn't feel the need to lose weight. I have been only peripherally envious of those naturally thin people, because they are just lucky. They never had to work at being thin, so I never felt the need to compare myself to them.

When we begin to make some progress both psychologically and physically in terms of weight loss, we inevitably begin to compare ourselves to those around us. Nevertheless, it is a mistake we must fight to avoid at all costs. Envy is an emotion that can only serve to harm us. Envy comes along this late on our emotional roller coaster because we are often too busy working on the more obvious emotions to consider this one a contender. It is something that is always there—an omnipresent character flaw. Yet most of us can override this emotion until we have dealt with other, more pressing, ones.

Only now that anger and frustration and other negative emotions have been examined and made to work in our favor can we begin to see envy for what it truly is—a negative emotional force that must be reckoned with. Let's look at the following questions to help us see how we can tame this emotion:

1. Who am I envious of?
2. What am I envious of?
3. What things in particular make me feel jealous toward another?
4. Does being jealous trigger other emotions?
5. Does being jealous bring any good into my life?

### Bonus Question: Do I truly have everything I need in order to make a real, concerted effort at this diet?

This is a harder question than you may think. This book provides you with the tools you will need to journey on this mind-body quest for thinness and health. When examining envy, you really need to question whether the things that make you envious will enable you to move toward your goal of better health. If they don't, you are wasting valuable time and energy. See envy for what it truly is—simply another road block. Destroy it and overcome it. I know you can do it.

**Mind-Body Medicines for Envy**
- Don't do all the right healthy things for the wrong reasons.
- The path of least resistance to doing the wrong thing is often the most chaotic.
- You are responsible to others, not for others; don't use them as an excuse.

**Recipes That May Help with Envy**
- Taj Mahal
- Fourth of July Chicken

# PART III

# THIN FOR GOOD:
# THE ANSWER
# TO YOUR
# DIETING PRAYERS

⊠

# CHAPTER 8

# The Guiding Principles of the Thin For Good Diet

And so we begin with a diet plan that will enable you to lose weight successfully, while remaining healthy and hunger free. There are many benefits to eating a healthy diet. It will give you more energy than you ever had before and it may even improve your sex life. And I promise you, as incredible as it might seem, you are going to have fun losing weight for the first time in your life.

There are certain guiding principles that apply to everyone. After you have finished reading this chapter, then go to chapter 9 if you are a woman or chapter 10 if you are a man, and find your appropriate stage.

## The Diet for You

1. Have you ever felt tired after eating or exhausted when you wake up in the morning?
2. In the afternoon, do you need a nap or crave carbohydrates and sweets?
3. Have you tried every diet in the world without success?
4. Do you believe that eating "right" means having cereal or fruit in the morning, salad for lunch, and pasta for dinner, and yet you still have those love handles, or even worse, feel crummy?
5. Do you know in your heart of hearts that thin people eat more food than you do?
6. Have you ever wondered whether it's just your metabolism that prevents you from losing the weight you want?
7. Have you ever binged on foods?
8. Do you experience mood swings?
9. Do you get irritable if you haven't eaten?
10. Do you know that others lose weight more easily than you?

If you answered Yes to any of these questions, then Thin For Good is the diet program for you. This diet is designed to minimize food cravings and alleviate many of those symptoms described above. This diet is not as restrictive as other low-carbohydrate diets, nor as boring as low-fat diets.

I have divided this chapter into several sections, with the main focus on the rules and structure of the diet.

## Let's Get Started

Let's begin with the *initiation phase* of the diet. This level of the diet is the strictest and it is the stage at which everyone who wants to lose weight should begin. This will be a good place to try to instill some of the discipline that is necessary if you want to remain thin after you've lost the weight you need or want to lose. Being on a diet will involve some work. You are going to have to make changes in the way you eat and you are going to have to establish new eating patterns—this often takes time. This is also the phase of the diet where you learn the mind-body medicines to help you understand some of the all-important mind games we play with ourselves and overcome some of the most difficult emotional roadblocks on the way to good health and losing weight.

The initiation phase of the diet is meant to last thirty days, although this depends on the amount of weight you need to lose. The more weight you have to lose, the longer this phase of the diet will last for you. It is entirely possible that this phase of the diet will last several months or longer. I am not here to fool you into thinking that no matter how much weight you may need to lose, whether it is 100 or just 10 pounds, the initiation phase of the diet will last the same amount of time. This is just not possible. Weight loss takes time, so don't try to rush things. You will get better results if you realize right from the beginning that you are in this to make positive and permanent changes, not just a quick fix.

The initiation phase of the diet is meant to help your body convert to a more efficient way of metabolizing food. Some people may experience a withdrawal syndrome as their bodies make this adjustment. This may consist of several days to even a week of feeling fatigued, irritable, and maybe even nauseous, depending on how addicted you were to your old style of eating. This is a normal reaction, so if you experience any of these symptoms during the first few days of the diet, bear with them and don't give up. They will go away. This is simply your body's way of making an adjustment to this new way of eating.

There's a good reason why you may experience some of these symptoms. Basically, what you're doing is changing what your body had been using as fuel—primarily sugar in one of its many disguises—and substituting protein, fat, and some complex carbohydrates, all much more efficient forms of energy, but ones that our bodies are no longer used to using.

In most cases, although you will probably feel some differences in your body, they will not be as extreme as the ones I've just described, and you will make the adjustment to this new way of eating without any noticeable discomfort.

Since I feel nutritional supplements are an important part of any diet program, please see chapter 19, the section for dieters, and use these as I have suggested.

## Foods to Eat in the Initiation Phase

Following are the allowable foods for anyone starting this diet. In the individual sections for women and men, I will divide the components into appropriate portions. Portion control need not be an issue for most people on this diet, as the portions are really quite generous and may well be larger than you are used to eating now. Nevertheless, I firmly believe that portion control must be learned in order to be a successful dieter and embark on your new nutritional lifestyle program. The truth is, it is not possible to eat as much food as you would like without suffering the repercussion of being overweight. Rest assured that you will not be measuring every morsel of food that goes into your mouth.

I believe that we will never be successful in our quest to be thinner unless we learn to control what we eat. Here is where the mind-body medicines can really help you. Recite them instead of reaching into the refrigerator. Or use their wisdom to help you see that it is not really the food that you want, but maybe something altogether different. Keep in mind that for every food category listed, there will be allowable portions mentioned in the individual chapters on sex and stage.

## Proteins

Proteins are the cornerstone of this diet. Many dieters still think they must stay away from this branch of the food chain if they are ever going to lose weight. This is not true. For one thing, protein can make a big difference in the way people feel by properly regulating the insulin response described in chapter 2.

Protein is important for many of the body's functions, including tissue growth, immune system regulation, muscular strength and tone, digestion, and the formation of hormones. Because of the differences in muscle mass between men and women, men will require more protein than women. These differences will be outlined in more detail in chapters 9 and 10.

Protein intake must be balanced with complex carbohydrates and fat in order to obtain a favorable insulin hormonal balance. Protein activates glucagon, the hormone that assists us in losing weight, building lean muscle mass, stabilizing energy levels, and controlling hunger.

Another advantage of eating protein is that when the amount of protein you ingest is raised in relation to the amount of carbohydrate ingested, a balance is achieved and your appetite is normalized. As a result, food cravings will disappear. Fat can also trigger leptin (a brain chemical) that tells us when we are full. Since healthy fat and protein play a large part in this diet, you will almost never be hungry if you follow the rules.

## Red Meats

Allowable red meats include beef, veal, lamb, pork, rabbit, venison, and other game animals.

For extra health benefits, I tell my patients some tips that I'll share with you. You need not follow these tips to maintain the integrity of the diet; they are just healthier suggestions.

- Trim the fat off the meat because most of the toxins and antibiotics the animal has consumed will be stored in its fat.
- Try to avoid processed meats. By this I mean luncheon or breakfast meats that have sugar, nitrates, or nitrites added. Most of these products have been cured in sugar, and most contain a chemical preservative that may be carcinogenic. I generally prefer turkey or roast beef, if you must eat from deli counters, as they are usually not changed much from their original form.

## Fish

Essentially, there are no limitations on fish. The fish permitted include, but are not limited to, tuna, salmon, swordfish, herring, pompano, whitefish, tilapia, cod, sole, bluefish, flounder, bass, and trout. Also permitted is all shellfish: scallops, shrimps, lobster, crab, conch, crawfish, abalone, squid, clams, and oysters, as well as calamari.

- I recommend that your fish not be farm raised unless you are familiar with the feeding practices that are used at the farm.
- Try to avoid or limit the amount of larger fish that you eat, such as tuna and swordfish, as well as shellfish, because they tend to contain higher levels of mercury, which may pose a health risk.
- Fish skin is perfectly acceptable. However, bear in mind that the fish will store toxins in the fat layer found in its skin. For health reasons, I prefer that you don't consume fish skin.
- Fish are very high in omega-3 fatty acids, which have been shown to have enormous health benefits. I recommend you consume as much of your protein from this category as you can. Because fish is so beneficial, I highly encourage these oils be taken in supplementation form. (See chapter 19 for more details.)

## Poultry

All poultry is allowed on the diet. This includes, but is not limited to, chicken, turkey, duck, cornish hens, pheasant, quail, and guinea hen.

- Avoid eating poultry skin, because that is where any toxins and antibiotic residue are stored.
- Dark meat has more fat than white meat. It is harder to get the proper balance you need between protein and fat when you consume too much fat. This is why I will often recommend that you use the white meat from poultry rather than the dark meat.
- The fats consumed while eating chicken are the natural saturated fatty acids.

## Eggs

Eggs are a marvelous form of protein. They have received bad press in the past few years, although they have recently been rehabilitated by mainstream nutrition researchers. Eggs, by themselves, do not raise your cholesterol. In fact, the yolk has a natural and very inexpensive cholesterol-lowering agent in the form of lecithin. Lecithin is also believed to raise the good cholesterol (HDL). Almost all of an egg's nutritional value is found in the yolk. Never eat whites without eating the yolk, and never eat egg substitutes. Rats that were fed only egg substitutes died from malnutrition.

If you purchase nothing else that's organic, please buy and eat only organic eggs. There is a significant difference in chemical composition between eggs that are conventionally raised and those that are organic. This simple and not much more expensive purchase makes eggs a great source of nutrition. Organic eggs contain omega-3 and omega-6 fatty acids in the beneficial ratio of 1 to 1. Commercial eggs, on the other hand, contain up to nineteen times more omega-6 than omega-3 fatty acids, making them much less healthy. It's not the cholesterol, but rather the poorly balanced fatty acid ratio that is the menacing culprit in eggs.

Another health tip is to try to always ensure that the egg yolk is thoroughly cooked. This will decrease your risk of contracting salmonella, which is rampant in commercially raised hens. This is something else you can avoid if you buy organic eggs. If the source of the hen is not contaminated with salmonella, then the egg won't be, either. Most organic farms do not harbor this bacteria, whereas most commercial farms do; that is one of the reasons why their chickens are fed antibiotics, and the organic ones are not.

## Cheese

All cheeses are permitted on this diet. These include both aged and fresh varieties. The only cheese I don't recommend is packaged American cheese—it really isn't cheese at all, but rather a "food product." Also, never use cheeses that are sold as low-fat. When the fat is removed, sugar or vegetable oil is added to the cheese to give it some taste. Try to avoid these if you can. Also, any aerosol cheese and any other cheese labeled as a "food product" should be avoided.

For all the proteins I've just described, there will be a section in both the male and the female chapters that will tell you how much of each you can consume, based on which stage you are in. *Also, please remember that there are no unlimited amounts of anything allowed on this diet.*

## Complex Carbohydrates

There are three kinds of carbohydrates: sugar, starch, and fiber. Sugar and starch, the simple carbohydrates, are easily digested by the body. Fiber, which includes bran and pectin, will pass through the body virtually intact. Fiber is also able to slow down the metabolism of simple carbohydrates when eaten together with them, forestalling the oversecretion of insulin.

Complex carbohydrates are the only carbohydrates allowed on the initiation phase of the diet. These include the low-carbohydrate vegetables, as well as higher-carbohydrate foods such as whole grains, whole cereals, beans, and legumes, in limited quantities.

The amount of complex carbohydrates permitted in this phase of the diet is determined by your stage and will be discussed in the appropriate chapter. Regardless, you should try to divide any allowable carbohydrates among your three meals, in order to achieve a proper balance.

This is a metabolically active diet. You cannot make up for straying from this diet in one day. Once your body has attained the metabolically active state of balanced insulin regulation, any deviation from your diet will cause a chemical shift, and it will take you approximately three days to recover.

### Vegetables

There are several variations on the vegetable theme. The first category is the lowest-carbohydrate salad vegetables, which are less than 10 percent carbohydrates. These include the green leafy vegetables like iceberg, romaine, Boston, and Bibb lettuces; escarole, endive, arugula, spinach, kale, and bok choy; as well as fennel, mushrooms, olives, celery, radishes, peppers, bean sprouts, and cucumbers. (This is not meant to be an exhaustive list; other forms of lettuces are also in this category.)

The second category of vegetables is between 10 and 25 percent carbohydrate. These include broccoli, cauliflower, eggplant, asparagus, turnips, tomatoes, avocado, snow pea pods, cabbage, scallions, onions, leeks, water chestnuts, zucchini, string beans, spaghetti squash, Brussels sprouts, artichoke hearts, okra, collard greens, and dandelion greens.

The third category of vegetables is the highest in carbohydrate content. They may even be considered starches or legumes. These include peas, corn, carrots, beets, parsnips, winter squashes such as butternut, buttercup, or acorn, white potatoes, and sweet potatoes. The ethnic vegetables, such as jicama, breadfruit, christophene, cassava, and plantains, to name a few, also fit in this category.

## Grains

Only complex grains are allowed on the diet. When choosing a bread or a grain product, always look for the word "whole" on the ingredient label. Most breads that are sold as wheat bread are just brown white bread, so don't be fooled into buying the wrong product. Look for products that say "whole oat," "whole wheat," or "whole rye" on the label.

Brown rice, which contains the fiber of the rice kernel, is also included in this category. White rice is not allowed because it is not a complex carbohydrate and is metabolized by the body in much the same way as sugar.

There are many other healthy grains, too. The alternative grains I recommend are amaranth, buckwheat (kasha), soy flour, kamut, teff, spelt, milo, millet, and quinoa. I know these may sound foreign to you, but many of them are commonly found in your local supermarket chains. If unavailable there, they can easily be found in health food stores.

Whole grain cereals are usually the hardest to find in the grocery stores. They contain the endosperm, germ, and fiber-rich bran of the grain. You may find the following table of some cereals helpful.

### Which Cereals Are Whole and Which Are Refined?

| Whole Grain | Mostly Refined |
|---|---|
| *Cold Cereals* | |
| Cheerios | Basic 4 |
| Granola or muesli | Corn flakes |
| Nutri-Grain | Frosted Flakes |
| Shredded wheat | Just Right |
| Total | Kix, Corn Pops |
| Wheat germ | Product 19 |
| Wheaties | Puffed Wheat |
| | Rice Krispies |
| | Special K |

| Whole Grain | | Mostly Refined |
|---|---|---|
| | *Hot Cereals* | |
| Oat bran | | Cream of rice |
| Oatmeal | | Cream of wheat (farina) |
| Quaker Multigrain | | Grits |
| Ralston High Fiber | | |
| Roman Meal | | |
| Wheatena | | |

Source: USDA Nutrient Database for Standard Reference, Release 11

## Pasta

Most familiar pastas are made from refined carbohydrates and hence are not permitted on the diet. That includes the Jerusalem artichoke pastas, the tomato pastas, and the like. They are all just as bad as "brown white bread" and are made to appear different simply to trick the consumer. There are whole wheat pastas on the market. You must check the food label. However, there are plenty of pasta alternatives these days. These include pasta made from spelt, kamut, soy, brown rice, quinoa, and even corn. Only if the pasta is made from a whole grain and it says so on the label is it allowed.

## Nuts and Seeds

Nuts and seeds are foods that have been overlooked in recent years. In large part, this is because they tend to be high in fat. That may be true, but they are also high in the good fatty acids, and many recent studies have shown them to be quite heart healthy.

However, some nuts are healthier than others. The first nut/seed category includes the ones I prefer: almonds, pecans, walnuts, and brazil nuts. Peanuts also could be included in this category, since most people consider them nuts although they are actually legumes. But many people are allergic to them, and they also contain a substance called aflatoxin, which may be harmful to some people. For these two reasons I don't like to include peanuts on the diet. However, many of my patients use peanut butter because they like it, and I even include it in many recipes (unsweetened, of course). Sunflower, pumpkin, and sesame seeds also fall into this first category.

The second category of nuts/seeds includes cashews and pistachios. These nuts/seeds are allowed in much smaller portions than the others because they are higher in carbohydrate. Macadamia nuts also fall into this second nut/seed category because of their higher fat content. They make a delicious snack—in moderation.

## Legumes

The legume category includes lentils, kidney beans, black beans, lima beans, fava beans, black-eyed peas, and navy beans. Bean products, such as tofu and tempeh, are also included in this category.

# Desserts

The only commercially available permissible dessert is a sugar-free gelatin product. However, there are many recipes in the back of this book for different types of desserts you can make yourself. It is possible to have desserts on this diet, but most of them you will have to make yourself from the allowable ingredients.

## Artificial Sweeteners

I do not favor the use of artificial sweeteners because of their strange chemical natures. But they are often a necessary evil, especially when it comes to dieting, and there are some that I feel are better than others.

These products comprise cyclamates, saccharin, acesulfame-K, aspartame, and the recently approved but not yet readily available sucralose, or trade name Splenda. Splenda is currently available in Canada and other countries and will be widely available in the United States in the early part of 2000.

Cyclamates have been taken off the market in the United States because of a cancer scare. Saccharin has also been relegated to second fiddle because of a cancer scare that has since been debunked. I believe saccharin is the safest of the artificial sweeteners.

Acesulfame-K is the poor relation in this field and is not used in too many products. Sucralose sounds incredibly promising. It is 600 times sweeter than sugar and is actually made from natural sugar that has been slightly chemically altered. Because it is made from sugar, you will be able to cook with it and it will not lose any of its sweetness. However, chlorine molecules have been added, and that doesn't sound healthy to me.

Currently, the most prevalent artificial sweetener in the world is aspartame. Aspartame is made of phenylalanine (one of the chemicals manufactured by the brain that acts as a neurotransmitter), aspartic acid, and methanol. Methanol, when metabolized, turns into formaldehyde, a chemical preservative. There have been many reports of adverse side effects from the use of this product, including gastrointestinal upset, headaches, rashes, depression, seizures, memory loss, blurred vision, blindness, slurred speech, and other neurological disturbances. For this reason, I would recommend avoiding any diet product that contains aspartame. Unfortunately, that is not always possible, since most diet products use it as a sweetener. I have even had to include it in some of my recipes. Anyone with PKU should also avoid this product, because of the phenylalanine.

There is a safe alternative to aspartame and other artificial sweeteners: stevia. Stevia is a plant found primarily in the rain forests of South America, but it is cultivated around the world. It contains no calories and is all natural. Most governments, including the United States and Canada, will allow this product to be sold only as a food supplement, and therefore it can be purchased in health food stores, but it is not allowed in food products, because it has not been widely tested in the United States.

## Condiments/Butter/Oils

Condiments permitted on this diet include: butter, olive oil, mayonnaise, lemon juice, vinegar, mustard, and most spices. Check the labels of combination spice preparations for sugar in any of its hidden forms. Catsup is not permitted on this diet due to its strong sugar content. And, because it is a trans fatty acid of the worst kind, margarine is strongly discouraged.

*Daily Allowances of Condiments for Men and Women in All Stages*

| | |
|---|---|
| Butter | 3 tablespoons |
| Olive Oil | unlimited |
| Mayonnaise | 3 tablespoons |
| Lemon Juice | 6 teaspoons |
| Vinegar | 4 tablespoons |
| Mustard | 4 tablespoons |

## Beverages

### Water

I believe water should be the beverage of choice for everyone. As we age, most of us become chronically dehydrated. This is because we are so used to going without something to drink that our body turns off our thirst mechanism. I often hear my patients tell me they are never thirsty. You should still have something to drink, anyway.

Water is crucial to the dieting process. It helps your body eliminate any toxins that may accumulate in the course of a day. It can also coax the residual water out of your cells. My patients who follow the water rule lose more weight than the patients who don't.

Water is essential to life. But it does more than quench your thirst. It helps regulate your body temperature, cushion your joints, remove toxins, maintain strength and endurance, protect organs and tissues, and carry nutrients and oxygen to every cell in your body. By the time you are actually experiencing thirst, you are mildly dehydrated. There are many subtle signs associated with dehydration, and I would bet that you experience some of these symptoms all the time without knowing why. These symptoms include: headache, fatigue, flushed skin, light-headedness, and dry mouth.

Certain studies have found that people who are dehydrated burn 3 percent less calories at rest than those who are not dehydrated. If you don't drink enough fluid, your body won't burn as many calories and it will take longer for you to lose weight. Therefore, I have a strict requirement for the amount of water that you must drink every day you are on this diet.

*You should be drinking the amount of water in ounces that your body weighs in kilograms.* A kilogram is 2.2 pounds. Divide your weight by 2.2, and that is the amount of water, in ounces, that you should drink each day. The more you weigh, the more water you should drink. For instance, if you weigh 220 pounds, divide 220 by 2.2 and get 100. If you weigh 220 pounds, you should drink 100 ounces of water per day. Eight glasses per day is not enough for most overweight people. The water may be tap, filtered, spring, bottled, or carbonated.

There are also two important conditions to this rule.

1. If you exercise, you need to add an additional 8 ounces of water for every 45-minute workout—16 ounces for running, tennis, or other high-intensity activities.
2. For every ounce of caffeinated beverage you drink, you need to drink 2 additional ounces of water.

Certain foods contain high levels of water. To determine how many ounces of water is in each of the foods listed below, simple multiply the weight of the serving by the percentage of water. For example, a 6-ounce serving of salmon contains 3.6 ounces of water. You can count the water in the food you eat as part of the daily requirement, should you choose to, but it is not critical to do so.

| Food | Percent Water |
| --- | --- |
| Lettuces of most kinds, zucchini, cucumbers | 95% |
| Asparagus, peppers, broccoli, cauliflower, cabbage, spinach, clams | 90% |
| Tofu, yogurt | 85% |
| Cottage cheese | 80% |
| Avocados, cod, eggs, ricotta, tuna | 75% |
| Brown rice | 70% |
| Skinless chicken | 65% |
| Salmon | 60% |
| Mozzarella cheese | 50% |
| Most other cheeses | 35% |

## Soda

I am not a big fan of soda. But if you must have it, diet soda is the only permissible kind of soda allowed on the diet. Soda sweetened with sugar or any sugarlike substance, such as fruit juice or barley malt, is not allowed. Diet sodas all use artificial sweeteners. In addition to its potential negative health implications, aspartame interferes with blood sugar metabolism, because it may be able to mimic the effect of sugar in the body, thereby causing insulin to be secreted, resulting in food cravings. This is the kind of metabolic behavior we are trying to avoid. That one simple thing can destroy the balance we are trying so hard to maintain. Too often, I have treated patients without any weight loss whose only mistake was drinking too much diet soda. Once they stopped all the aspartame, they began to lose weight. Enough reason not to drink it.

## Coffee/Tea

Coffee and tea should be avoided. The decaffeinated versions are better, but I still don't like my patients to have these items. The only beverages in this category I do recommend are herbal teas.

There are two reasons for my disapproval. The first is that caffeine, by causing insulin to be secreted, may have a blood sugar destabilization effect and lead to cravings. The second reason is that in the processing procedure, many manufacturers use petroleum-based products, which may be dangerous. There are also potentially harmful tannins, found more often in tea than in coffee, that may have a negative effect on your health.

I believe these products to be unhealthy, but by consuming them you will not be going off the diet and the diet's integrity will still be maintained. I offer these health tips so you may get the most benefit out of your new nutritional lifestyle program.

No grain beverages are allowed.

## Milk

There are two categories of milk. The first includes regular milk and its close cousins, skim milk and lactose-free milk. The drinking of milk is not allowed because of all the sugar that's in it. Skim milk and lactose-free milk are also forbidden on the initiation diet, because they have the same amount of sugar per serving as regular milk. If you need to use something in your coffee, I recommend using cream. Cream can also be used in recipes as a thickening agent for sauces. Never use nondairy creamer—the reason is as obvious as the label on the carton. Yogurt is included in this category. It is not allowed in the initiation phase of the diet.

The second category includes soy milk, rice milk, and non-cow animal milks. If these are to be used, they must be unsweetened. Many of these milks, especially rice milk, can be sweeter even than regular milk. Check the labels and look for the unsweetened variety. Only those are permissible, and in extremely limited quantities on the initiation diet.

## Alcohol

Alcohol is strictly limited in this diet program, even eliminated in some stages. The first category includes scotch, bourbon, and all the other brown liquors. The second category includes white liquors, such as vodka and gin. The third category includes wines and beers.

# Fruits

All fruits are not created equal. As in many other food groups, fruits can be divided into different categories. This is done according to sugar and water content in the fruit. For the most part, fruits are comprised of a simple sugar. They do have fiber in the form of pulp, and that is what makes the actual fruit acceptable but not fruit juice.

Fruit juice is nothing more than colored sugar water. It is not healthy and its use is one of the biggest food myths perpetuated in our society today. Most fruit juices have more sugar per serving than soda. In fact, your body does not know the difference between soda and fruit juice.

The first category of fruits includes melons such as cantaloupe, honeydew, crenshaw, and watermelon; and berries, such as raspberries, strawberries, and blueberries.

The second category includes grapefruits, peaches, plums, and nectarines.

The third category includes apples, kiwis, and oranges.

The fourth category includes the tropical fruits, such as banana, mango, papaya, and guava.

There is a world of food possibilities out there. We all get so caught up in our daily routines we forget that things exist outside of our own little world. This concept also applies to food. Many patients can't believe all the foods that are available to them on this diet.

My hope is that this diet will help expand your culinary horizon and help you see that you don't have to deprive yourself to be thin—but you do have to think yourself thin! Diet is not about deprivation, it's about a way of life. This diet program will help you begin to get your mind and body into the proper alignment that it needs in order to lose weight.

The foods I have mentioned in this chapter are not meant to be an exhaustive list. Instead, I want you to go out and create your own diet from the foods mentioned here. In the next two chapters, you will see where the restrictions lie. After reading them, you can use this list to make a diet that is suitable to you. Each of us has different tastes, and with my diet you will be able to plan your meals accordingly—and enjoy eating your way to slimness.

Over the years of observing patients on this diet, I have noticed certain common pitfalls. Here are some simple ways to avoid them:

1. The initiation phase does not contain any sugar of any kind.
2. Avoid diet products unless they specifically have no sugar. They usually are very high in simple carbohydrates and sugars.
3. Please don't be fooled by the word "sugarless." That simply means that a product contains no white sugar, but there may be sugar in one of its other disguises. Check the label carefully.
4. Please be aware that cough syrups, chewing gum, gum drops, and food made specifically for diabetics all contain sugar, and should be avoided.

THE ELEVEN EMOTIONAL LEVELS OF EATING
# LEVEL 8: BOREDOM

This is a killer of an emotion and one that many people use to stop their new nutritional lifestyle program. Have you ever said, "This diet is boring," "The way I am eating is boring," or any of a million of these excuses? Know that it is your mind's way of overcompensating for your body's desires. Boredom comes late on our road to being thin and healthy because there were a lot of emotions that needed to be handled before we could ever get here. And by this point, the initial excitement of starting a diet has begun to wear off. But some people use boredom as an excuse not to start dieting. They already have the preconceived notion that this diet will be more boring than the way they eat now.

This is an emotion that needs to be transformed, or at the very least handled in a way that allows you the greatest freedom. Isn't that what it's all about? We paint ourselves into these little boxes of can and cannot. In terms of dieting, no matter what diet you follow, there are hundreds of food choices, yet somehow we can still allow ourselves to think that our diet is boring. I would bet that if you wrote down what you ate even before starting a diet, you would find many of the ways you were eating were repetitious—fast food or pasta, for example, night after night. Eating the same foods over and over again is boring. *The boredom we experience is all in our heads.* Be creative to avoid boredom. You have the ability to make the diet not boring or, at the very least, to experience your diet in a nonboring way.

Let's look at some questions to help you determine the role boredom plays in your dieting life:

1. What makes me bored?
2. Who makes me bored?
3. When am I most free to make my own decisions?
4. Who makes most of the food decisions in my household?
5. What foods make me the most bored?

## *Bonus Question: Have I ever used boredom as an excuse to go off a diet? If so, why? If not, why not?*

The focus of this may surprise you. Is it really boredom or your perception of boredom? How does boredom play a role in our food decisions? Should it? I tell my patients it should not. Boredom is what each and every one of us makes it out to be. Otherwise, what interests you would always interest me and vice versa. That is never the case and will not be the case with food, as well as in life. You have the power to turn boredom into something positive. Some people would even look on the routine of certain foods as empowering. It is all in your mind, and you have the power to make of it what you want.

**Mind-Body Medicines for Boredom**
- Expectations about weight-loss outcomes affect results.
- We must constantly overcome our nature to eat the wrong foods.
- Inject certainty into the dieting situation.

**Recipes That May Help Alleviate Boredom**
- Sunday on a Wednesday Eggs
- Top-Hat Burger

CHAPTER 9

# The Thin For Good Initiation Phase for Women

At long last, here is a diet designed specifically for women. But going even further, it is also a diet that is designed for the many stages in a woman's life—a unique, simple, and fun way for you to lose weight.

One of the biggest complaints I hear from couples who are on different diets is that it takes too much time to prepare the different foods. That will not happen with this diet plan. There will be slight differences in your meal structure, depending on your stage, but nothing too complicated, as the foods from which to choose are the same.

This chapter will be divided according to the various stages. If you find that this diet is not working as well as you would have hoped, retake the quiz in chapter 6, making sure you answer each question truthfully to ensure that you are in the right stage. If, after retaking the quiz, you find that you have started in the right stage, then move to the next higher stage, as that is usually a stricter one. If this still doesn't work for you, later on in this book I will describe other scenarios that may explain why you may be having difficulty losing weight.

If you are a vegetarian, read chapter 11.

Keep in mind when looking at the portion amounts that the portion sizes are listed as uncooked weights. Another important thing that applies to all women, no matter the stage, is the water rule. You must drink, in ounces, your weight in kilograms. This is easy to figure out. All you have to do is to take your weight in pounds and divide it by 2.2. That is your weight in kilograms and the amount of water you need to drink every day in ounces. For example, if you weigh 154 pounds, divide this number by 2.2 and you get 70. You need to drink 70 ounces of water per day while on this diet.

By following this diet program, you can become thin for good. More important, you will decrease some of the major risk factors for heart disease, such as triglyceride and total cholesterol levels; osteoporosis; breast cancer, by decreasing the excess amount of estrogen stored in fatty tissue; and type II diabetes—simply by losing weight. The diet may even help with many menopausal symptoms. All of these positive health changes have occurred in my patients as a result of this program. They can happen for you, too, if you follow the entire program.

In Part IV of this book is a 30-day meal plan that transcends all the stages (even for men), so you will have a general idea of the rich diet you can expect to be on for the coming months. This will also include the mind-body daily doses for a complete approach to losing weight.

This chapter is going to discuss what and how much you can eat, by category of food, for each different stage. A more detailed list of food choices from all the categories of food may be found in chapter 8. From the foods and the restrictions I am about to mention, you will be able to choose your own meals and make this a unique diet plan that perfectly suits you. Also, don't forget to try the nutritional supplements for the dieter as outlined in chapter 19.

Let's begin.

# The Beginner

## Proteins

In most cases, each protein section will be divided into three basic categories.

- All category 1 foods are limited to 8 ounces per day.
- All category 2 foods are limited to 12 ounces per day.
- All category 3 foods are limited to 16 ounces per day.

This categorization is done according to the amount of fat found in the foods. As you will see, these general rules do not apply to eggs and cheese.

As a general rule, you are allowed a maximum portion of 6 ounces of protein for breakfast, 10 ounces for lunch, and 14 ounces for dinner. This does not mean that you have to consume this amount in any given day, only that you can if you'd like.

### Red Meats

*Category 1:* includes beef and pork.
*Category 2:* includes veal, lamb, and rabbit.
*Category 3:* includes venison and many of the other game animals.

Remember to *trim the excess fat* from the meat.

### Processed Meats

These meats include bacon, Canadian bacon, sausage, ham, and most lunch meats. They are allowable on the diet in the following ways: 2 ounces of breakfast meats and 4 ounces of luncheon meats per day. Roast beef is permissible as a category 1 red meat, because deli roast beef is usually just roasted beef and nothing else. Deli turkey is usually just turkey and is permissible as in the poultry category.

### Fish

*Category 1:* shellfish. This includes shrimps, scallops, octopus, squid, clams, oysters, conch, mussels, crab, and lobster.

*Category 2:* includes herring, pompano, and whitefish.

*Category 3:* includes tuna, salmon, sardines, scrod, trout, cod, flounder, sole, sardines, trout, mackerel, and others.

### Poultry

There are only two categories of poultry.

*Category 1:* the dark meat, such as thighs, legs, and neck, as well as all duck parts.

*Category 2:* the light meat, such as breasts and wings.

### Eggs

Eggs are permitted without restriction, and you should never eat the white of the egg without eating the yolk.

### Cheeses

*Category 1:* cheeses that are hard and aged, including Swiss, cheddar, muenster, and mozzarella, as well as Brie, and any other cheese not mentioned in category 2 below. Up to 4 ounces of these are allowed each day.

*Category 2:* cheeses of the fresh variety, including farmer's cheese, pot cheese, cream cheese, cottage cheese, and ricotta. These are limited to 4 ounces each day.

## Complex Carbohydrates

### Vegetables

*Category 1:* essentially salad vegetables, such as all types of lettuce, fennel, mushrooms, olives, bok choy, celery, radishes, peppers, bean sprouts, and cucumbers. Up to 6 cups of lightly packed greens are permitted each day.

*Category 2:* includes broccoli, cauliflower, eggplant, cabbage, scallions, onions, leeks, water chestnuts, zucchini, string beans, spaghetti squash, Brussels sprouts, and artichoke hearts. Up to 1 cup permitted each day.

*Category 3:* includes peas, corn, carrots, beets, parsnips, winter squashes such as butternut, buttercup, or acorn, white potatoes, and sweet potatoes, and the ethnic vegetables such as jicama, breadfruit, christophene, cassava, and plantains. These are permitted in a very limited amount: ¾ cup three times each week.*

### Grains

Please make sure these are the complex grains that I've described in chapter 8. They are permitted in the amount of a ¾ cup serving, or 1 slice of whole grain bread, three times each week. This includes pasta, as long as it is a whole grain variety.*

### Nuts and Seeds

*Category 1:* almonds, pecans, walnuts, brazil nuts; sunflower, pumpkin, and sesame seeds. Up to 1 ounce allowed each day.

*Category 2:* Macadamia nuts, cashews, and pistachios. These are not allowed.

### Legumes

Legumes, including lentils, kidney beans, black beans, lima beans, fava beans, black-eyed peas, navy beans, tofu, and tempeh, are permitted up to a ¾ cup serving three times each week.

## Desserts

The only dessert I recommend in this phase of dieting, unless it is a recipe from this book or one similar to it, is a sugar-free gelatin product.

## Condiments

See chapter 8.

## Beverages

Water is the preferred drink for this diet according to the rules stated in chapter 8. The water may be tap, filtered, spring, bottled, or carbonated.

Anything flavored with sugar, including fruit juice, is not allowed.

### Soda

Regular soda is not permitted.

Diet soda: no more than 12 ounces per day. This includes any other beverage that may be artificially sweetened.

---

*You may have *either the grains or the category 3 vegetable*s on those three days each week. This does not mean that you may have these six days each week, only three. It is an and/or category, not an and/and category.

**Alcohol**

*Category 1:* the brown liquors, such as scotch and bourbon. Up to 4 ounces permitted three times each week.

*Category 2:* the white liquors, such as gin and vodka. These are not permitted.

*Category 3:* wine and beer. These are not permitted.

**Milk**

*Category 1:* Heavy cream is allowed up to 2 tablespoons per day; otherwise not permitted.

*Category 2:* Unsweetened soy or rice milk is allowed up to 4 ounces three times a week; otherwise not permitted.

**Fruit**

*Category 1:* melons, such as cantaloupe, honeydew, and watermelon. These are permitted up to a ½ cup serving three times a week.

*Category 2:* grapefruit, peaches, plums, and nectarines. These are not permitted.

*Category 3:* apples, kiwis, and oranges. These are not permitted.

*Category 4:* other tropical fruits such as banana, pineapple, mango, and guava. These are not permitted.

As you can see, this is not a very restrictive diet. What this diet does, however, is to take into account all the different types of food, then balances them in your diet. This will always be the key to long-term success.

## Diet for the Young Woman

Women of this stage have a different awareness of themselves and their bodies. They know what looks good on them, what makes them happy, and are more secure with their position in life. It is during this period that women are coming into the prime of their lives, and not just sexually. This is an enviable position to be in, yet many women are truly suffering from a lifetime of eating the wrong way.

Everything and everyone you take care of may be the biggest obstacle to taking care of yourself. Isn't it ironic that at the time in your life when you are supposed to be in your prime, you're overweight and fatigued? My diet will allow you to get back into shape so that you can enjoy these years with health and vitality. Don't get angry anymore or frustrated—my diet allows you to get even.

As far as dieting goes, this is a time when things begin to get a little rough. You may have begun to accept some of the seemingly inevitable weight gain that occurs with age, yet it doesn't have to happen if you just follow these simple guidelines.

You will need to keep chapter 8 handy as a reference guide. That chapter explains in more detail the various types of foods by category. This section will tell you the amounts of food from each category that you may have. Then you can fashion your own diet according to what you like to eat.

## Proteins

As a general rule, you will be allowed a maximum portion of 4 ounces of protein for breakfast, 8 ounces for lunch, and 12 ounces for dinner. These are maximum daily amounts. Don't feel as if you have to eat this amount every day. This amount can take the form of any of the foods that follow. Generally, each protein section will be subdivided into three basic categories.

- All category 1 foods are limited to 6 ounces per day.
- All category 2 foods are limited to 10 ounces per day.
- All category 3 foods are limited to 14 ounces per day.

This categorization is made according to the amount of fat found in the foods. As you will see, these general rules do not apply to eggs and cheese.

### Red Meats

*Category 1:* beef and pork
*Category 2:* veal, lamb, and rabbit
*Category 3:* venison and other game animals

Excess fat should be trimmed from all meats.

### Processed Meats

I would prefer that you avoid processed meats, but if you can't, breakfast meats are permissible up to 2 ounces, and luncheon meats up to 3 ounces, each day. Breakfast meats include bacon, sausage, Canadian bacon, etc. Lunch meats include all the deli meats except roast turkey and roast beef, as they are generally just roasted meats. Roast beef is included in red meat category 1, and turkey is included in poultry category 2.

### Fish

*Category 1:* shellfish, including shrimps, scallops, lobster, crabs, oysters, clams, mussels, conch, octopus, and squid
*Category 2:* herring, pompano, whitefish
*Category 3:* tuna, salmon, flounder, sole, cod, scrod, swordfish, mackerel, and all fish not included in any of the above categories

**Poultry**

Poultry is divided into only two categories, by type of meat.

*Category 1:* dark meat such as legs, thighs, and neck, as well as all duck parts

*Category 2:* white meat, such as breasts and wings

**Eggs**

Up to six eggs a day are permitted. Never eat the white of the egg without the yolk, as the yolk is the most nutritionally important part of the egg.

**Cheese**

*Category 1:* hard, aged cheeses such as Swiss, cheddar, blue, Brie, and Monterey Jack, etc.; any cheese not in category 2 below. These cheeses are limited to 4 ounces each day.

*Category 2:* the soft, fresh cheeses such as cottage cheese, farmer's cheese, pot cheese, cream cheese, and ricotta. Up to 3 ounces allowed each day.

## Complex Carbohydrates

**Vegetables**

*Category 1:* salad vegetables, including all lettuces, kale, fennel, mushrooms, bok choy, celery, radishes, peppers, bean sprouts, and cucumbers. You may have up to 4 cups each day of loosely packed greens.

*Category 2:* lower-carbohydrate vegetables, including broccoli, cauliflower, eggplant, asparagus, turnips, cabbage, tomatoes, snow pea pods, leeks, water chestnuts, zucchini, string beans, spaghetti squash, artichoke hearts, okra, collard greens, dandelion greens, and Brussels sprouts. Up to ½ cup allowed each day.

*Category 3:* peas, corn, carrots, beets, parsnips, winter squashes such as butternut, buttercup, or acorn, white potatoes, sweet potatoes, and the ethnic vegetables such as jicama, breadfruit, christophene, cassava, and plantains. These are permitted in a ½ cup serving twice each week.*

**Grains**

Grains must only come from the following list: brown rice, amaranth, teff, kamut, spelt, milo, millet, quinoa, and any other grain that includes the word "whole" on the label. Pasta may be included in this category, as long as it is one of the whole grain varieties. Grains are permitted in the amount of a ½ cup serving twice each week, or 1 slice of whole grain bread twice each week.*

---

* Please keep in mind that you may have either the Category 3 complex carbohydrate vegetables *or* the grains twice a week, not both.

### Nuts and Seeds

*Category 1:* almonds, pecans, walnuts, and Brazil nuts; sunflower, pumpkin, and sesame seeds. These are allowable up to 1 ounce a day.
Roughly, this translates into 10 nuts. This may not sound like a lot,
but if you give the nuts half a chance to be digested and the oil to be
absorbed, you will find that this amount is surprisingly filling.

*Category 2:* pistachios, cashews, and macadamia nuts. These are not permitted in this phase of the diet.

### Legumes

The legumes include lentils, kidney beans, black beans, lima beans, fava
beans, black-eyed peas, navy beans, tofu, and tempeh. They are permitted
up to a ½ cup serving three times each week.

## Desserts

There are several dessert options to be found in the recipe section of this
book. You may also be able to create variations of your own. However, the
only commercially available dessert permitted is sugar-free gelatin. This
may be consumed in unlimited quantities—just be aware that it is sweetened
with aspartame.

## Condiments

See chapter 8.

## Beverages

Water is a dietary requirement. You must drink your body weight in
kilograms, translated into ounces of water, each day. The water may
be tap, filtered, spring, bottled, or carbonated.

Anything flavored with sugar, including soda and fruit juice, is not allowable.

Diet soda is permitted up to 12 ounces a day as a recommended maximum. This includes any other beverage that is flavored with artificial
sweeteners.

### Alcohol

*Category 1:* The brown liquors, such as scotch and bourbon, are permissible up to 2 ounces twice a week.

*Category 2:* The white liquors, such as gin and vodka, are not permitted.

*Category 3:* Wine and beer are not permitted.

**Milk**

Category 1: Heavy cream is permitted up to 2 tablespoons per day; otherwise not permitted.

Category 2: Unsweetened soy or rice milk is allowable up to 4 ounces twice per week.

## Fruit

Category 1: melons and berries. Up to a ½ cup serving allowed twice each week.

Category 2: grapefruits, peaches, plums, and nectarines. They are not permitted.

Category 3: apples, kiwi, and oranges. They are not permitted.

Category 4: tropical fruits, such as bananas and mangoes. They are not permitted.

This diet is relatively easy for this phase of your life. If you have any difficulty, please jump into the next category because that is the strictest category, and you may fare better being somewhat stricter. The final call as to which stage you will be in is up to you and how well you do. The guidelines I offer here are the ones I use in my practice and that work for the majority of the patients I see.

# The Perimenopausal/Menopausal Woman

The perimenopausal/menopausal woman has the most difficulty losing weight, which generally has to do with hormones. Perimenopause begins much earlier than we ever used to believe. The hormonal changes that occur start as early as the late thirties. This may explain some of the subclinical symptoms many women begin to experience at this time of their lives, such as memory loss, not feeling as together as they once did, not functioning as sharply as they once did, and many other similar things that most women just ignore. Then, one day, you miss a period and you've got a name for what you have. Keep chapter 8 available as a handy reference guide as to the types of foods you can have. The amounts of the foods are discussed below.

## Proteins

As a general rule, you will be allowed a maximum portion of 2 ounces for breakfast, 4 ounces for lunch, and 8 ounces for dinner. These are maximum allowable daily amounts, and this entire amount does not need to be consumed on a daily basis in order to maintain the integrity of the diet. This protein can take the form of any of the foods that follow.

Most protein sections will be divided into three basic categories.

- All category 1 foods are limited to 3 ounces each day.
- All category 2 foods are limited to 6 ounces each day.
- All category 3 foods are limited to 8 ounces each day.

The categorization is made according to the amount of fat in each category of food. These general rules do not apply to eggs or cheese, which have their own set of rules.

### Red Meats

*Category 1:* beef and pork
*Category 2:* veal, lamb, and rabbit
*Category 3:* venison and other game animals

The excess fat should be trimmed from all meats.

### Processed Meats

You may have 1 ounce of breakfast meats such as bacon, Canadian bacon, sausage, and ham steak and 2 ounces of lunch meats, such as salami, bologna, mortadella, and ham. Roast beef from a deli is generally just roasted meat and is therefore permissible as a red meat category 1. Turkey from the deli is usually just roasted turkey and may be considered a category 2 poultry.

### Fish

*Category 1:* shellfish, including shrimp, scallops, lobster, crab, oysters, clams, mussels, conch, octopus, and squid
*Category 2:* herring, pompano, and whitefish
*Category 3:* tuna, salmon, cod, scrod, mackerel, haddock, halibut, trout, sardines, swordfish, flounder, sole, etc.

### Poultry

This section is divided into two categories, by type of meat.

*Category 1:* dark meat, which includes legs, thighs, and necks. This also includes all duck parts.
*Category 2:* white meat, which includes breasts and wings

Remove the skin for health reasons.

### Eggs

The maximum number of eggs that you ought to eat each day is three. Remember, never eat the egg white without eating the egg yolk. The yolk is where all the natural omega-3 fatty acids are located.

**Cheeses**

> *Category 1:* hard cheeses such as Swiss, cheddar, Brie, Roquefort, muenster, etc; any cheese not listed in category 2 below. These are limited to 2 ounces each day.
>
> *Category 2:* the soft cheeses, including cream cheese, cottage cheese, pot cheese, farmer's cheese, and ricotta. They are allowed up to 1 ounce each day, enough to use as a snack.

## Complex Carbohydrates

**Vegetables**

> *Category 1:* all the leafy salad vegetables, such as the various types of lettuce; and fennel, mushrooms, olives, bok choy, celery, radishes, peppers, bean sprouts, and cucumbers. Up to 3 cups of lightly packed greens are permitted each day.
>
> *Category 2:* green beans, broccoli, cauliflower, eggplant, asparagus, tomatoes, avocado, olives, snow pea pods, cabbage, scallions, leeks, water chestnuts, zucchini, string beans, spaghetti squash, artichoke hearts, okra, collard greens, dandelion greens, and Brussels sprouts. These are allowed up to ½ cup each day.
>
> *Category 3:* peas, corn, carrots, beets, parsnips, winter squashes, white and sweet potatoes, and ethnic vegetables such as jicama, breadfruit, christophene, cassava, and plantains. These are not permissible.

**Grains**

Grains must be of the complex variety. Look for the word "whole" on the label or choose from the following groups: brown rice, amaranth, buckwheat, kamut, spelt, teff, quinoa, milo, and millet. Up to a ½-cup cooked serving, or 1 slice of whole grain bread, permitted once each week. This category includes pasta, as long as it is whole grain and in the permissible amount.

**Nuts and Seeds**

> *Category 1:* almonds, pecans, walnuts, Brazil nuts; sunflower, pumpkin, and sesame seeds. Up to ½ ounce, roughly the equivalent of 5 nuts, is allowed per day. They will make an excellent snack. If you think five nuts is nothing, just give them a chance to work their magic on your digestive tract before you reach for more. If you still feel hungry after five nuts, wait five minutes—I assure you your feeling of hunger will disappear.
>
> *Category 2:* macadamia nuts, cashews, and pistachios. These are not permissible.

### Legumes

These include lentils; kidney, black, lima, and fava beans; black-eyed peas; and tofu and tempeh. These are allowed up to a ½-cup serving a week.

## Desserts

A portion as described in the menu section of the desserts in this book is allowed. The only commercially prepared dessert that is allowable is a diet gelatin product. You may have unlimited amounts of that product.

## Condiments

Please refer to chapter 8 for full details on condiments.

## Beverages

Water is the beverage of choice. It is imperative and a dietary rule that you must drink the number of ounces of water each day that is the number of kilograms you weigh. (See chapter 8.) The water may be tap, filtered, spring, bottled, or carbonated.

Anything flavored with sugar is not permissible. That goes for fruit juice and soda as well.

Diet soda: 12 ounces of diet soda, or another artificially sweetened beverage, is permissible per day.

### Alcohol

*Category 1:* brown liquors, such as scotch and bourbon. They are not permitted.

*Category 2:* white liquors, such as vodka and gin. They are not permitted.

*Category 3:* Wine and beer. They are not permitted.

### Milk

*Category 1:* Heavy cream is allowed up to 1 tablespoon per day; otherwise not permitted.

*Category 2:* includes soy, rice and non-cow animal milks. These are not permitted.

## Fruit

*Category 1:* Melons and berries are allowed up to a ¼ cup serving each week.

*Category 2:* includes peaches, plums, nectarines, and grapefruit, and they are not permitted.

*Category 3:* includes apples, kiwis, and oranges, and they are not permitted.

*Category 4:* includes the tropical fruits such as bananas, mango, and papaya, and they are not permitted.

There it is, the definitive diet for the perimenopausal/menopausal woman. I know it's not easy, but it's probably not as hard to follow as you think. There are really many foods allowed on the diet—the portions are just more limited than in any other stage or sex category. You will still be able to eat a well-balanced diet and be able to go on this diet with friends and family with only minor modifications.

## The Postmenopausal Woman

This diet is not as restricted as the one for perimenopausal/menopausal women. At this stage in your life, menopause has generally occurred and your body is slowly beginning to compensate for the hormonal imbalances. If you are taking hormonal replacement therapy, then you should do the perimenopausal/menopausal diet. In my clinical experience I have found that hormonal replacement therapy makes it difficult for a woman to lose weight.

Despite the decreased level of activity that most women will experience in this stage, if you follow the simple guidelines I've set forth, you will be able to easily shed those pounds that may have been accumulating for years.

Please keep in mind that the following food choices are to tell you the amount of each different type of food you may have. All the individual selections of the different types of foods per category are listed in chapter 8.

### Proteins

As a general rule, you are allowed a maximum portion of up to 3 ounces for breakfast, 6 ounces for lunch, and 10 ounces for dinner. This does not mean that you need to eat this entire amount if you are not hungry. Generally, each protein section will be subdivided into three basic categories.

- All category 1 foods are limited to 4 ounces per day.
- All category 2 foods are limited to 8 ounces per day.
- All category 3 foods are limited to 10 ounces per day.

The foods are categorized according to their fat content. These general guidelines will apply to all proteins, except cheese and eggs.

#### Red Meats

*Category 1:* beef and pork
*Category 2:* veal, lamb, and rabbit
*Category 3:* venison and the other game animals

Trim the excess fat as much as you can to eliminate any potential toxins the animal may have stored.

### Processed Meats
The breakfast meats, including sausage, bacon, Canadian bacon, and ham, must be limited to 1 ounce each day. The lunch meats, which include salami, bologna, boiled ham, etc., must be limited to 3 ounces each day. Turkey and roast beef from most delis will just be roasted meats, and are allowable up to the limits for red meat (roast beef) and poultry (turkey).

### Fish
> *Category 1:* shellfish, including shrimp, scallops, clams, oysters, mussels, crab, lobster, conch, octopus, and squid
> *Category 2:* herring, pompano, and whitefish
> *Category 3:* tuna, salmon, cod, swordfish, flounder, cod, scrod, mackerel, halibut, trout, sardines, sole, haddock

### Poultry
This section is divided into only two categories.

> *Category 1:* dark meat, such as legs, thighs, and neck, and all duck parts
> *Category 2:* white meat, such as breasts and wings

Remove the skin from poultry.

### Eggs
Up to five eggs a day are permitted. Never eat the white of the egg without the yolk. The yolk is the most nutritionally important part of the egg.

### Cheese
> *Category 1:* the hard, aged cheeses such as Swiss, cheddar, blue, Brie, Monterey Jack; any cheese not listed in category 2 below. These cheeses are limited to 3 ounces each day.
> *Category 2:* the soft, fresh cheeses such as cottage cheese, farmer's cheese, pot cheese, cream cheese, and ricotta. These are allowed up to 2 ounces each day.

## Complex Carbohydrates
### Vegetables
> *Category 1:* salad vegetables, including all the various types of lettuce, kale, fennel, mushrooms, olives, bok choy, celery, radishes, peppers, bean sprouts, and cucumbers. Up to 4 cups of loosely packed greens are allowed each day.

*Category 2:* asparagus, green beans, broccoli, eggplant, cauliflower, cabbage, snow pea pods, scallions, onions, leeks, water chestnuts, zucchini, string beans, spaghetti squash, artichoke hearts, okra, collard greens, dandelion greens, and Brussels sprouts. These are allowable up to ½ cup a day.

*Category 3:* peas, carrots, corn, winter squashes (butternut, buttercup, or acorn), beets, parsnips, white potatoes, sweet potatoes, and the ethnic vegetables such as jicama, christophene, breadfruit, cassava, and plantains. These are permitted in a ½-cup serving once a week.*

### Grains

Grains must only be of the whole grain variety. Check your labels. Whole grains include: brown rice, kamut, spelt, quinoa, teff, amaranth, buckwheat, milo, and millet. Pasta may be included in this category, as long as it is one of the whole grain varieties, and is in the proper amount. Grains are permitted in the amount of a ½-cup serving, or 1 slice of whole grain bread, twice a week.*

### Nuts and Seeds

*Category 1:* almonds, pecans, walnuts, Brazil nuts; sunflower, sesame, and pumpkin seeds. These are allowed up to ½ ounce each day, or roughly 5 nuts. This may not sound like a lot, but if you give the nuts a chance to be digested and the oil to be absorbed, you will find that this amount is surprisingly filling.

*Category 2:* cashews, pistachios, and macadamia nuts; not permitted in this phase of the diet.

### Legumes

This category includes lentils; kidney, fava, black, white, navy, and lima beans; black-eyed peas; tofu and tempeh. These are allowed up to a ½-cup serving twice a week.

## Condiments

Please refer to chapter 8 for full details on condiments.

## Desserts

There are several dessert options to be found in the recipe section of this book. You may also be able to create variations of your own. However, the only commercially available dessert is sugar-free gelatin, which may be consumed in unlimited quantities. Be careful of your aspartame consumption.

---

*This is an and/or category coupled with the category 3 vegetables above. You are allowed either category 3 vegetables or the grain servings each week, not both.

## Beverages

Water is a dietary requirement. You must drink, each day, the number of ounces of water that is the number of kilograms you weigh. The water may be tap, filtered, spring, bottled, or carbonated.

Anything flavored with sugar, including soda and fruit juice is not allowed.

Diet soda, or any other drink that may be sweetened with artificial sweeteners, is permissible up to 12 ounces a day.

### Alcohol

*Category 1:* the brown liquors, such as scotch and bourbon, are allowed up to 2 ounces a week.

*Category 2:* the white liquors, such as gin and vodka, are not permitted.

*Category 3:* wine and beer are not permitted.

### Milk

*Category 1:* heavy cream is allowed up to 2 tablespoons per day; otherwise not permitted.

*Category 2:* unsweetened soy or rice milk is allowable up to 2 ounces twice per week.

### Fruit

*Category 1:* melons and berries are allowed up to a ½-cup serving each week.

*Category 2:* grapefruits, peaches, plums, and nectarines are not permitted.

*Category 3:* apples, kiwis, and oranges are not permitted.

*Category 4:* tropical fruits, such as bananas, mangoes, papayas, and pineapples, are not permitted.

There are so many healthy foods you can eat on this diet and still lose weight. You will almost never feel hungry, and you will almost never experience a food craving. The reason for this is that if you follow this diet correctly, you will have been able to find the correct balance for you. Once that balance is attained, losing weight—and even more important—maintaining that weight loss becomes easy.

Chapter 10 is for the men in your life. You may read it, if you wish, or you can simply skip to chapter 12 to read about the forever phase. However, don't skip the Eleven Emotional Levels of Eating found at the end of chapters 10 and 11.

# THE ELEVEN EMOTIONAL LEVELS OF EATING
## LEVEL 9: RELIEF

Relief is another emotion I see in patients as something that is really transitional. It is the beginning of positive emotions—and don't you feel kind of strange! It is almost as if we don't know how to handle anything that may make us feel relatively good. That may be a new experience for you. And you know what, it's perfectly all right to feel a little strange, a little awkward, a little out of character. You feel that way because you are. It is probably going to be a new experience for you to feel lighter, healthier, and thoroughly prepared for the future. It may the first time in your life you have ever successfully completed a diet and known that the future is yours—that the weight is never going to go back on.

These can be empowering emotions, but they can also have a destabilizing effect on the progress you have made so far. At this point, most dieters are relieved that they have managed to successfully navigate another diet and lose weight yet again. With this diet, most dieters are relieved to know that they will probably never have to go on another diet again because this will work for them. There is a sense of relief and a sense of accomplishment. However, with every good emotion comes the responsibility to maintain that feeling.

My advice in this situation is to allow yourself to feel the relief. Sit back and enjoy the sensation, even if it is only for a moment or two. Try not to let the old demons crawl back into your consciousness, as they will be trying so desperately to do. Take a stand, feel relieved, know that you have done some great work to get to this point, and try not to predict the future. If you can do this, the next emotional level is yours to keep.

Here are the questions I give my patients to help them determine how they generally handle situations in which they feel relieved:

1. When do I feel a sense of relief?
2. Who makes me feel relieved?
3. Does feeling relieved make me feel comfortable?
4. What other emotions come up for me when I feel relieved?
5. Have I ever felt a true sense of relief from anything in my lifetime?

### Bonus Question: What set of actions do I take when I feel relieved?

This is the most important aspect to the sense of relief. Most people have some level of anxiety or heightened sense of awareness when they are dieting. They are more diligent and pay more attention to what is going on in their daily lives, especially in terms of eating. The real key is what to do once this edginess is no longer a part of your life—once you've mastered the diet and its eating principles and achieved the weight loss you have wanted. Most of us will let our guard down, and in dieting land that usually means a binge coming along. That doesn't have to happen if you explore some of the reasons why this may happen to you. Although most patients experience this sense of relief, what separates the most successful from the nominally successful is how they navigate this emotional level.

### Mind-Body Medicines for Relief

- Inject certainty into the dieting situation.
- The path of least resistance to do the wrong thing is often the most chaotic.
- You must have more than a momentary commitment to being thinner.

### Recipes That May Help with Relief

- Rosemary-Scented Zucchini Soup
- Louisville Oeufs

# The Thin For Good Initiation Phase for Men

Finally, here's a diet designed exclusively for men, one that allows you to eat real food. I've always wondered, as I'm sure you have, too, how diet experts can expect men to eat salads, pastas, and other stuff and expect you to feel satisfied? Sure, you probably would lose weight, but more than likely you'd feel hungry, deprived, and miserable all the time. How could you ever stay on a diet like that? How many times has your wife or girlfriend expected you to follow a diet she found in some women's magazine? Sure, 3 ounces of salmon might satisfy her appetite, but what about you?

The diet described in this chapter is different from the one I give to women because a diet for men must also take into consideration the various changes that occur in a man's life as he ages. It is not just women whose hormonal balance changes as they age. It happens to men, too. These hormonal changes affect our energy level, moods, stamina, sex drive, and most important, our ability to maintain or lose weight.

The diet found in this chapter takes all this into consideration as well as the fact that it's not possible for you to lose weight on the same diet as a man who is in a different stage of life. That's why I developed the stages. And despite the fact that these diets are different, they are not so different—with a few slight adjustments you will be able to diet with your wife, or a partner, who is following my diet too.

From my experience, most men want to lose weight for health rather than cosmetic reasons. My diet takes those concerns into consideration. The diet outlined in this chapter will help you reduce your chances of suffering from many of the leading health problems affecting men today—heart disease, diabetes, and prostate cancer, to name only a few.

Eliminating some of the major risk factors for heart disease, which is the leading health concern for men, includes lowering your total cholesterol, raising your HDL or good cholesterol, decreasing your triglyceride level, lowering your homocysteine level, and—less obvious but no less important—lowering your weight. All these positive health changes have occurred in many of my patients, and they may occur for you when you follow this diet program. Your chances of getting adult onset, type II diabetes will also decrease because your weight will go down and you will be eating markedly less sugar.

The initiation phase will be divided into three separate male stages, based on my clinical experience and on the research done on the metabolism of men. You only need to read the stage that applies to you. If you are having difficulty losing weight with the diet stage that you have selected, then go back to the quiz in chapter 7 and be certain that you have answered all the questions correctly and honestly. If you still get the same score and land in the same category, then try the next category up and see if that works for you. If you are still having difficulty losing weight, there may be another process occurring in your body. I will be describing many of these trouble areas in a later chapter, so don't give up. Also, it is important to remember that the mind-body exercises play an enormous role in this diet. Don't discard these or think you don't need them. Make sure you understand them and the rules of the diet that applies to your stage and I am almost certain you will have no difficulty losing the weight you desire, getting the energy you would like, and having your sex drive back where it belongs.

In the coming sections, I will outline the additional rules for each male stage. Chapter 8 contains a more detailed food list. You should refer to that chapter as we go along. From the foods and the restrictions I am about to mention, you will be able to choose your own foods to make this a unique diet plan that suits you and your lifestyle, whether it is active or not so active. I think it is important for people to be able to outline their own meal plans rather than have me do it for them, as I don't always know what people like. In Part IV of this book is a 30-day menu plan that transcends all the stages, for men and women, so that you will have a general idea of the rich diet that you can expect to be on for the coming months. This will also include the daily mind-body doses so that you truly have the most comprehensive strategy for weight loss.

Another important thing that applies to all men, no matter the stage, is the water rule. You must drink, in ounces, your weight in kilograms. This is easy to figure out. All you have to do is to take your weight in pounds and divide it by 2.2. That is your weight in kilograms and the number of ounces of water you need to drink on any given day. For example, if you weigh 176 pounds, divide this number by 2.2 and you get 80. You would need to drink 80 ounces of water per day while on this diet.

Vegetarians should skip to chapter 11. Don't forget to include the nutritional supplements to help with your Thin For Good Diet Program as outlined in chapter 19.

# The Beginners

Men in this category have the easiest time with the weight loss part of this diet program. No matter what the reason, many men in this stage have begun to gain weight. It may seem as if it happens overnight, but believe me, it doesn't, and neither will the weight loss. Nevertheless, if you follow all the guidelines for your stage, you can probably expect to lose, on average, 3 to 6 pounds per week in this phase of the diet.

## Proteins

The maximum allowable portion you can have is 6 ounces of protein for breakfast, 14 ounces for lunch, and 20 ounces for dinner. This is not to say you must eat that much food. Just know that it is available to you if you need it. In most cases you will probably not need that much food, as this diet is very satisfying and you won't be as hungry as you usually are.

The protein category is divided into groups of foods, which are then subdivided into categories. Each category is based on the amounts of fat present in the food and so the amount of fat you will be eating will vary each day, depending upon the type of protein you will be consuming.

- All category 1 protein foods are allowed up to 12 ounces each day.
- All category 2 foods are allowed up to 16 ounces each day.
- All category 3 foods are allowed up to 20 ounces each day.

These portions are more than you will probably need. Also, you can mix the types of protein you eat. But you must not exceed the maximum, which is 40 ounces in total each day. There is a different set of rules for eggs and cheese.

### Red Meats

*Category 1:* beef and pork
*Category 2:* veal, lamb, and rabbit
*Category 3:* venison and other game animals

Trim the excess fat from all meat as much as possible, because the animal stored all of its toxins, and any antibiotic it may have consumed, in its fat.

### Processed Meats

All breakfast meats, which includes bacon, Canadian bacon, sausage, and ham, should be limited to 3 ounces each day. All lunch meats such as bologna, salami, ham, mortadella, etc. must be limited to 8 ounces each day. Roast beef and turkey from the deli are generally just roasted meats and are therefore permissible as is stated in their respective categories, provided they do not have any sugar added to them.

### Fish

*Category 1:* shellfish, including clams, oysters, mussels, lobster, shrimp, scallops, crab, octopus, conch, and squid
*Category 2:* herring, pompano, and whitefish
*Category 3:* tuna, swordfish, salmon, sole, halibut, cod, mackerel, flounder, haddock, trout, and sardines

### Poultry
This section has only two categories.

*Category 1:* dark meat, such as thighs, legs, and necks, and all parts of duck
*Category 2:* white meat, such as breast, and wings

Eliminate all the skin that you can for health reasons; animals store toxins in the fat found in the skin layer.

### Eggs
Eggs are unlimited. Never eat the whites without the yolk. You should look for eggs that have a higher amount of omega-3 fatty acid than omega-6, and organically grown eggs come closer to the all important 1:1 ratio than the average commercially produced egg.

### Cheeses

*Category 1:* hard or aged varieties, including Swiss, cheddar, muenster, Monterey Jack, and anything not mentioned in category 2. These are permitted up to 6 ounces each day.
*Category 2:* the fresh or soft varieties of cheese, including cottage cheese, pot cheese, farmer's cheese, cream cheese, and ricotta. These are allowed up to 4 ounces each day.

## Complex Carbohydrates
### Vegetables

*Category 1:* salad vegetables, including the varying types of lettuce and spinach, kale, fennel, mushrooms, olives, bok choy, celery, radishes, peppers, bean sprouts, and cucumbers. Up to 6 cups of lightly packed greens are permitted each day.
*Category 2:* lower-carbohydrate vegetables, such as eggplant, onion, tomato, broccoli, cauliflower, asparagus, cabbage, leeks, scallions, water chestnuts, zucchini, string beans, avocado, spaghetti squash, turnips, artichoke hearts, okra, collard greens, and dandelion greens. These are permitted up to 1 cup each day.

*Category 3:* peas, corn, winter squash, carrots, beets, parsnips, potatoes (white or sweet), and the ethnic vegetables, such as jicama, breadfruit, cassava, plaintains, and christophene. These are permitted up to a ½ cup cooked serving three times each week.*

## Grains

These must be eaten in the form of complex grains, as described in chapter 8. Examples include brown rice, amaranth, teff, buckwheat, kamut, spelt, milo, millet, and quinoa. This also includes whole wheat, whole oat, whole rye, and any grain you are familiar with as long as the label reads "whole." They are permitted up to a ½ cup cooked serving three times each week; or 1 slice of whole grain bread three times each week. Pasta, if it is of the whole grain variety and limited in amount, is included in this category.*

## Nuts and Seeds

*Category 1:* pecans, almonds, walnuts, Brazil nuts; sunflower, pumpkin, and sesame seeds. These are allowed up to 1 ounce, which roughly translates into 10 nuts each day. That is a satisfying amount if you eat them slowly. Try to eat only half the allowable nuts at any one sitting, and allow the beneficial oils to coat your stomach. Wait for at least five minutes, and this will be enough to satisfy your hunger. This way, you can save the other half for later in the day.

*Category 2:* cashews, macadamia nuts, and pistachios. These are not permitted.

## Legumes

Examples of these include navy, pinto, fava, white, and kidney beans; black-eyed peas; tofu and tempeh. These are permitted up to a ¾ cup cooked serving three times each week.

## Desserts

There are many desserts available to you, but only choose from the ones listed in the recipe section of this book, or similar ones that you may create yourself. In those offered at the end of the book, I have listed the serving size that would be suitable for any dieter. The only commercially available dessert allowed is sugar-free gelatin. You may have as much of this dessert as you would like, but be careful of the amount of aspartame.

---

*You are permitted to eat either the grains or the category 3 vegetables three times a week, not both. You can alternate as well by having, for example, a grain one night and category 3 vegetables two nights, or whichever mix you prefer.

## Condiments

Please refer to chapter 8 for a full listing of the allowable condiments.

## Beverages

Drinking the right amount of water is the only steadfast rule that must be followed to the letter. You must drink the number of ounces of water equal to your weight in kilograms each day. The water may be tap, filtered, spring, bottled, or carbonated.

Anything flavored with sugar, which includes soft drinks and fruit juice, is not permitted.

Diet soda and any other artificially sweetened beverage is permissible up to 12 ounces a day.

### Alcohol

*Category 1:* the brown liquors, such as scotch and bourbon. They are permissible up to 4 ounces three times per week.

*Category 2:* the white liquors, such as gin and vodka. These are not permitted.

*Category 3:* wine and beer. They are not permitted.

### Milk

*Category 1:* heavy cream is allowed up to 2 tablespoons per day; otherwise not permitted.

*Category 2:* unsweetened soy or rice milk is allowed up to 2 ounces three times per week.

## Fruit

*Category 1:* melons and berries—up to ½ cup serving allowed three times each week.

*Category 2:* grapefruits, plums, nectarines, and peaches are not permitted.

*Category 3:* apples, oranges, and kiwis are not permitted.

*Category 4:* bananas, mango, papaya, guava, and pineapple are not permitted.

That's all there is to it. It's not as hard as you thought, and certainly this diet can satisfy a man's appetite. Following this diet plan is going to increase your energy and improve your life in many ways. You don't have to follow a specific menu every day. Instead, you may make up your own menu. You may eat many of the foods you like and still lose weight painlessly. It is possible to put together many exciting meals from these choices. It is even easy to eat out. If you prefer following a set menu, you may do this with the one offered at the beginning of Part IV.

# The Weekend Warrior

Metabolically, this is the time in your life when the levels of testosterone are starting to decline at the rate of about 1 percent per year. This decline sets the stage for some of the problems associated with dieting. Our metabolism slows down because our muscle mass starts to decline, because we probably aren't exercising as much as we used to, and because of the decline in testosterone production.

My diet will help your body overcome some of these obstacles that affect dieting by giving you the correct balance that you need at this stage of your life. This will very likely be your first experience with dieting, because for the first time in your life you are probably beginning to worry about your health, something those who care about you have probably been doing for you for years. Now, *you* are concerned. The guidelines that follow were formulated with your stage of life in mind. Chapter 8 explains in full detail all the different foods that are available in all the separate categories. From the guidelines mentioned below, you will be able to set your own diet and choose your own foods. If you are interested in a sample menu, one follows in the next part of this book.

## Proteins

You will be allowed as a maximum daily portion 4 ounces of protein for breakfast, 10 ounces for lunch, and 16 ounces for dinner. However, this does not mean that you have to eat this much protein in a day. Each protein category is divided into three sections, according to the amount of fat found in each type of food.

- All category 1 foods are allowed up to 6 ounces each day.
- All category 2 foods are allowable up to 10 ounces each day.
- All category 3 foods are allowable up to 12 ounces each day.

These are larger amounts than I just mentioned, because some people will prefer different types of protein in any given day, and that is all right, as long as you stay within the maximum daily allowable portions. These rules do not apply to eggs and cheese.

### Red Meats

*Category 1:* beef and pork
*Category 2:* lamb, veal, and rabbit
*Category 3:* venison and other game animals

Trim the excess fat for an especially healthy serving of red meat.

## Processed Meats

Breakfast meats, including bacon, Canadian bacon, sausage, and ham, are limited to 2 ounces each day. Lunch meats include salami, bologna, mortadella, ham, etc., and are limited to 6 ounces each day. Roast beef and turkey from the deli are usually just roasted meats. If they are, and have had no sugar added, their limits are defined in the individual sections—red meat for roast beef, poultry for turkey.

## Fish

*Category 1:* shellfish, including oysters, clams, mussels, lobster, crab, shrimp, scallops, conch, squid, and octopus
*Category 2:* herring, pompano, and whitefish
*Category 3:* tuna, salmon, swordfish, mackerel, cod, flounder, haddock, and sardines

## Poultry

This section has only two categories.

*Category 1:* dark meat, such as the legs, thighs, and necks, and all duck parts
*Category 2:* white meat, such as breasts and wings

Keep this category extra healthy by avoiding the skin of the poultry.

## Eggs

Eggs are limited to 6 each day. Remember this caveat: Do not eat the whites of the egg without eating the yolk.

## Cheeses

*Category 1:* hard cheeses, such as Swiss, muenster, cheddar, Brie, or any cheese not mentioned in category 2. These are limited to 4 ounces each day.
*Category 2:* fresh cheeses, such as cottage cheese, farmer's cheese, pot cheese, cream cheese, and ricotta. These are allowed up to 2 ounces each day.

## Complex Carbohydrates

### Vegetables

*Category 1:* salad vegetables, such as all types of lettuce; spinach, kale, fennel, mushrooms, olives, bok choy, celery, radishes, peppers, bean sprouts, and cucumbers. These are allowed up to 4 cups of lightly packed greens each day.

*Category 2:* lower-carbohydrate vegetables, including cauliflower, turnips, tomato, onion, leeks, scallions, cabbage, snow pea pods, water chestnuts, zucchini, spaghetti squash, Brussels sprouts, avocado, collard greens, and dandelion greens. These are allowed up to a ¾ cup cooked serving each day.

*Category 3:* Please refer to chapter 8 for a listing. Examples include peas, corn, carrots, beets, parsnips, winter squashes, and potatoes; and the ethnic vegetables, such as jicama, christophene, plantains, cassava, and breadfruit. These are allowed up to a ½ cup cooked serving once each week.*

### Grains

These must be only complex grains. These include whole wheat, whole oat, whole rye—any grain as long as the word "whole" appears on the ingredient list. Other examples include brown rice, amaranth, teff, buckwheat, kamut, spelt, milo, quinoa, and millet. Pasta may be permitted in this category, provided that it is of a whole grain variety, and in the correct amount. These grains are permitted up to a ¼ cup cooked serving twice each week; or 1 slice of whole grain bread twice each week.*

### Nuts and Seeds

*Category 1:* pecans, walnuts, almonds; sunflower and sesame seeds. These are allowed up to ½ ounce each day. This roughly translates into 5 nuts each day. I know this doesn't sound like a lot, but this amount can be very satisfying. Nuts and seeds have oils in their chemical makeup that are beneficial in terms of health. Also, fat takes longer to digest and decreases your hunger. Give the oils in the nuts about five minutes to start working before you reach for more food. According to the latest research, the fats in this category are quite heart healthy.

*Category 2:* macadamia nuts, cashews, and pistachios. They are not permitted.

### Legumes

These are permitted up to a ½ cup cooked serving twice each week. Examples include navy, pinto, and fava beans, lentils, kidney beans, black beans, lima beans; black-eyed peas; and tofu and tempeh. Please refer to chapter 8 for a discussion on which legumes are allowable.

---

*You are permitted either the grain or the category 3 vegetables, not both. This is important to keep in mind at all times. You may have one category one night and the other another night, for a total of twice each week maximum.

## Desserts

Aside from those desserts described in the recipe section of this book, or similar ones you may devise, there are really no permissible commercially prepared desserts, except sugar-free gelatin. You may have as much of this as you would like, but remember to watch your intake of aspartame.

## Condiments

Please see chapter 8 for a full discussion of condiments.

## Beverages

There is one hard and fast rule that you must follow in order to stay on this diet. You must drink, each day, the number of ounces of water that is the same number as your weight in kilograms. This helps to get rid of bodily toxins, and it also helps fill you up, so you won't become so hungry. The water may be tap, filtered, spring, bottled, or carbonated.

Soda or anything that is sweetened with sugar, including fruit juice, is not allowed.

Diet soda or any beverage that is artificially sweetened is permissible up to 12 ounces each day.

### Alcohol

*Category 1:* the brown liquors, such as scotch and bourbon. They are permissible up to 2 ounces three times a week.

*Category 2:* the white liquors, such as gin and vodka. These are not permissible.

*Category 3:* wine and beer. These are not permissible.

### Milk

*Category 1:* heavy cream is permitted up to 2 tablespoons per day; otherwise not permitted.

*Category 2:* unsweetened soy or rice milk is permitted up to 2 ounces twice each week; otherwise not permitted.

## Fruit

*Category 1:* melons and berries are permissible up to a ¼ cup serving twice each week.

*Category 2:* grapefruit, plums, nectarines, and peaches. These are not permitted.

*Category 3:* apples, kiwis, and oranges. These are not permitted.

*Category 4:* the tropical fruits, such as bananas, mangoes, guava, pineapples, and papayas. They are not permitted.

As you can see, this can be a satisfying way to lose weight. You may eat many of the foods you love—maybe not in the quantity you would like, but at least you're not eating "rabbit food." As a result, given the number of food choices, this can be a relatively painless way to lose weight. This is the perfect diet to help you trim down and truly get back into the shape you think you are in.

## The Experienced Male

If you are a man at this stage of life, you are probably looking forward to retirement, while at the same time starting to realize that you are not going to live forever. Maybe your wife is beginning to nag you to slow down and learn to enjoy the golden years. Maybe your sex life isn't as great as it used to be. Many of your friends are starting to have their first heart attacks. When you sit around at your weekly poker games, the talk is about your cholesterol levels, how many times you wake up to pee at night, or your PSA.

This is the time in most men's lives when we seriously start to get concerned about our health. Is it too late to do something about it? Probably not. As far as I'm concerned, it is never too late to start a good diet and exercise regimen.

I'm going to help you now with the diet part, because if you are like most men, you've probably either never had to worry about your weight or, if you had a weight problem, you probably never decided to do anything about it until now. So let's begin!

Keep in mind that what will follow are the allowable amounts of food in each category of food. The types of food in those categories are given in detail in chapter 8, so I recommend you keep that chapter handy as a quick reference.

### Proteins

You are allowed as a maximum daily amount 3 ounces of protein for breakfast, 8 ounces for lunch, and 14 ounces for dinner. This does not mean you need to eat the entire amount. The amount of fat consumed in these foods depends on several factors, and that is why the protein section is divided into three separate categories based on the amount of fat.

- All category 1 foods are allowable up to 6 ounces each day.
- All category 2 foods are allowable up to 10 ounces each day.
- All category 3 foods are allowable up to 12 ounces each day.

These are higher amounts than the daily total, depending on which type of protein you may wish to consume in any given day. There will be a different set of rules for eggs and cheeses.

## Red Meats

*Category 1:* beef and pork
*Category 2:* veal, lamb, and rabbit
*Category 3:* venison and other game animals

Trim the excess fat from all meat to ensure the maximum health benefit.

## Processed Meats

These are the breakfast meats and many of the lunch meats. Breakfast meats include bacon, Canadian bacon, ham, and sausage. Lunch meats include salami, ham, mortadella, bologna, etc. Breakfast meats are limited to 1 ounce each day; lunch meats are limited to 4 ounces each day. The lunch meats exempt from this set of stipulations are turkey and roast beef, as they are generally just roasted meats. They are permissible according to their respective categories, provided they don't contain sugar. Always check the label.

## Fish

*Category 1:* shellfish, including crab, lobster, shrimp, scallop, mussels, clams, oysters, conch, squid, and octopus
*Category 2:* herring, pompano, and whitefish
*Category 3:* tuna, salmon, swordfish, mackerel, sardines, flounder, sole, halibut, cod, scrod, bluefish, dolphin, tilapia, and all other types of fish not mentioned in the first two categories.

## Poultry

This section is divided into two categories.

*Category 1:* dark meat, such as legs, thighs, necks, and all duck parts
*Category 2:* light meat, such as breasts and wings

Avoid the skin to get the optimum health benefits.

## Eggs

Up to 3 eggs are permitted each day. Never eat the egg white without the egg yolk.

## Cheeses

*Category 1:* hard and aged cheeses, such as cheddar, Swiss, Brie, Roquefort, Monterey Jack, or any cheese not mentioned in category 2. These are limited to 2 ounces each day.
*Category 2:* fresh cheeses, such as cream cheese, pot cheese, farmer's cheese, cottage cheese, and ricotta. These are allowable up to 1 ounce each day.

## Complex Carbohydrates

### Vegetables

*Category 1:* leafy salad vegetables, such as all lettuce, spinach, kale; fennel, mushrooms, olives, bok choy, celery, radishes, peppers, bean sprouts, and cucumbers. These are permissible up to 3 cups of lightly packed greens each day.

*Category 2:* lower-carbohydrate vegetables, including green beans, asparagus, leeks, tomatoes, onions, cabbage, scallions, broccoli, cauliflower, eggplant, turnips, avocado, snow pea pods, water chestnuts, zucchini, spaghetti squash, Brussels sprouts, artichoke hearts, okra, collard greens, and dandelion greens. These are permitted up to a ½ cup cooked serving each day.

*Category 3:* includes beets, parsnips, winter squashes, potatoes, peas, corn, carrots, and other starchy vegetables. These are not permitted.

### Grains

These must be the complex grains as described in chapter 8. These include brown rice, amaranth, buckwheat, kamut, teff, spelt, milo, millet, and quinoa. Of course, more recognizable grains such as wheat and oat are also included in this category, provided the label describes them as "whole." Pasta is included here, as long as it is of the whole-grain variety. Grains are permitted up to a ¼ cup cooked serving each week; or 1 slice of whole-grain bread each week.

### Nuts and Seeds

*Category 1:* pecans, almonds, walnuts; sunflower and sesame seeds. These are permitted up to ½ ounce per day. Roughly translated, that means 5 nuts. I know that doesn't sound like a lot, but consider it a snack. If you eat them slowly and allow the oils of the nut to coat your stomach, giving them five minutes to work their magic, you will find your hunger will be satisfied.

*Category 2:* cashews, pistachios, and macadamia nuts. They are not permitted.

### Legumes

These include lentils, kidney beans, black beans, lima beans, fava beans, black-eyed peas, and navy beans. Bean products such as tofu and tempeh are also in this category. These are not permitted.

## Desserts

Choose from the dessert choices in the recipe section of this book. You may be able to come up with some similar creations of your own. The only allowable commercially available dessert is sugar-free gelatin, and you may have as much of this as you like, but be cautious of the amount of aspartame you are eating.

## Condiments

Please refer to chapter 8 for a full listing.

## Beverages

> You must consume, each day, the number of ounces of water that is the number of your weight in kilograms. The water may be tap, filtered, spring, bottled, or carbonated.
>
> Anything flavored with sugar is not allowed, and that includes soda and fruit juice.
>
> Diet soda or anything artificially sweetened is allowed up to a total of 12 ounces each day.

### Alcohol

> *Category 1:* scotch, bourbon, and other brown liquors. They are not permitted.
>
> *Category 2:* gin, vodka, and other white liquors. They are not permitted.
>
> *Category 3:* wine and beer are not permitted.

### Milk

> *Category 1:* heavy cream is allowed up to 2 tablespoons per day; otherwise not permitted.
>
> *Category 2:* soy milk, rice milk, and other non-cow animal milks; these are not permitted.

## Fruit

> *Category 1:* melons and berries. They are not permitted.
>
> *Category 2:* grapefruits, peaches, plums, and nectarines. They are not permitted.
>
> *Category 3:* apples, kiwis, and oranges. They are not permitted.
>
> *Category 4:* tropical fruit, such as bananas, guava, pineapples, mangoes, and papayas. They are not permitted.

As you can see, this can be an easy diet to follow, because there are not that many categories of food that are entirely eliminated. All you need to do is to determine your stage in life. Please use the quiz truthfully. Don't place yourself in a certain stage because you fancy yourself being in that category—that will only hurt your chances for true success with this program.

Take full advantage of the mind-body program I will outline for you. This is a definite edge you will have over most other dieters. The mind-body medicines will undoubtedly help you as they have helped me and many of my patients lose weight when they thought it was impossible.

If you adhere to the guidelines, you should find yourself losing weight soon, and you will also help eliminate many of the risks for the most common health problems that affect men.

Part IV lists a sample 30-day menu, and the all important mind-body program.

# THE ELEVEN EMOTIONAL LEVELS OF EATING
## LEVEL 10: JOY

Finally, you have made it to this level and the most positive emotion. You may be happy with the progress you've made or you may be happy with how you feel, or even how you look—or with all three. By this point you have achieved something worth shouting about, and celebrating. This is what you have been working for, whether it has taken months, weeks, or even years.

But still, isn't there that nagging feeling that there's something wrong? Do you believe that if it feels this good, something bad is about to come along and ruin it? This is the way many dieters turn something extremely positive into a negative. The other way joy can be turned into a negative is using feelings of elation to do something that may affect the integrity of your diet—for example, deciding that you have been so good, a piece of cake won't hurt a bit, will it?

Why sabotage yourself? Why think the worst? For most of us with a weight problem, these *feelings* may be inevitable. After all, hasn't the weight always gone back on? Doesn't someone always try to sabotage you?

Be content with the joy you are feeling. Allow that to be the positive energy it's meant to be. Allow some happiness to filter through your brain with the message that being thinner and healthier may be a good thing, even if it means having to change some of the ways you have always led your life. Joy can be exciting, but it may also lead to fear. Knowing this may make it easier to avoid the backsliding. Here are some questions that may help you see what role joy plays in your life:

1. What makes me happy?
2. Who makes me happy?
3. What foods have always equaled happiness in my life?
4. What things make me glad to be alive?
5. Who makes me glad to be alive?

### Bonus Question: Do I ever allow myself to experience joy or happiness for any length of time?

The amount of time you can stand feeling joyful and what other emotions this joy brings up for you is the definite driving force behind the use of this emotion to help you lose weight and attain a healthier lifestyle. You can do it, you just have to know that it may be uncomfortable. Step into the unknown and learn to experience the joy that follows as a result.

**Mind-Body Medicines for Joy:**

- No pain, no gain.
- If the reward is any good, you've got to earn it.
- You are in this dieting game, play it for all it's worth.

**Recipes I Associate with Joy:**

- White Gazpacho
- Mini Sour Cream Cheesecakes

# CHAPTER 11

# Thin for Good for Vegetarians

Susan, twenty-three, came to my office at the suggestion of many of her friends. They had all finished college and were beginning their new lives in the big city. Like most young women in their age group, they were extremely interested in their health but were utterly confused about what to eat and what they should avoid. They wanted to do the right thing and stay healthy, but with all the confusing information that was available they just didn't know how. The parent of one of the girls in the group had been my patient. She had lost 65 pounds, was feeling better than she ever had and wanted her daughter to experience the same great benefits. That young woman did particularly well, losing those 5 pounds every young woman wants to lose, and in the process she was able to work out longer, stay out later, and generally feel great. She recruited all of her friends to see me, too.

Susan was the last holdout because she was a vegetarian and couldn't see how a high-protein diet would ever fit into her lifestyle. I promised not to try to convert her into a meat eater, and she agreed to give it a try. After two weeks, she came bounding into my office with tons of energy and couldn't believe how changing her diet could make her feel so much better so quickly. She wasn't even aware that she had been feeling unwell. Oh, and she lost 12 pounds in the process. She could not have been happier.

Vegetarianism is probably not a topic that you thought would be included in a book of this kind. After all, I advocate a high-protein diet, which usually means lots of meat, meat products, poultry, fish, and not much else. However, in my years of practice, I have seen many patients who had been vegetarians their entire lives and wanted to stay that way. I needed to devise a program that would be suitable for them, so I created their own special diet. The rules in this chapter apply only to vegetarians and should not be mixed and matched with any of the other types.

These guidelines apply to both male and female vegetarians regardless of their stage in life. I have found the program to be effective for most vegetarians, so there is no gender differentiation in this chapter.

I created this special diet program for vegetarians for two main reasons. The first is I didn't want to exclude a significant segment of the population from receiving the benefits of a high-protein diet. The second reason is that I am truly horrified by what most North Americans believe to be a vegetarian lifestyle.

A majority of vegetarians in North America believe a vegetarian diet should consist of bread and pasta, a little soy, some veggies, and not much else. This is entirely wrong. In fact, a diet that consists primarily of bread and pasta is unhealthy. The truth is, most people don't realize that there are wonderful nonanimal sources of protein.

This special vegan diet is not for the armchair vegetarian, but for those who do not eat any animal products at all, not even eggs or cheese. A variation on this diet is for those vegetarians who do eat cheese and eggs, also known as lacto-ovo vegetarians. I believe this is a healthier way of being a vegetarian, because cheese and eggs are great sources of protein.

## The Water Rule

This rule applies to all vegetarians, too. You must drink, in ounces, your weight in kilograms. This is easy to figure out. All you have to do is to take your weight in pounds and divide it by 2.2. That is your weight in kilograms and the number of ounces of water you need to drink in any given day. For example, if you weigh 132 pounds, divide this number by 2.2 and you get 65. You would need to drink 65 ounces of water per day while on this diet.

## Diet for the Vegetarian

### Proteins

If you are a complete vegan, you are allowed as a maximum daily portion 6 ounces of protein for breakfast, 10 ounces for lunch, and 12 ounces for dinner. If you are a lacto-ovo vegetarian, you are allowed 4 ounces of protein for breakfast, 8 ounces for lunch, and 10 ounces for dinner. This does not mean you have to consume all the protein that's allowed, but it's there if you need it to satisfy your hunger.

Protein can be found in many nonanimal sources. This includes whole cereal grains, beans and bean products, and nuts and seeds. These allowable foods will be categorized, examples of foods from each category will be listed, and a daily allowable portion of each will be outlined for you, so all you need to do is to follow along.

#### Beans and Bean Products

This includes adzuki, broad, kidney, black turtle, pinto, lima, and mung beans; peas (although peas are legumes, I include them in this category to make it easier), soybeans, black-eyed peas, chickpeas, lentils, natto, tempeh, and tofu. Of these, tofu has the least amount of available protein per serving, believe it or not.

> *Category 1:* adzuki, mung beans, soybeans, tofu, chickpeas, and natto. These are allowed up to 16 ounces each day.
> *Category 2:* all the rest. These are allowed up to 4 ounces each day.

### Nuts and Seeds

> *Category 1:* almonds, pecans, walnuts, Brazil nuts, and peanuts (these are really legumes, but as most people consider them nuts, I place them here to eliminate any confusion. Please see chapter 8 for a warning on peanuts). These are allowed up to 2 ounces each day.
> *Category 2:* cashews and pistachios. These are allowed up to 1 ounce each day.
> *Category 3:* macadamia nuts. They are allowable up to ½ ounce each day.

Please note that 1 ounce of nuts is approximately 10 nuts. Don't go overboard—this may not sound like a lot, but nuts have the ability to satisfy your hunger rather quickly. Even with just 10 nuts, I tell my patients not to eat them all at one sitting, because they are that satisfying if you eat them slowly and give the natural oils in the nuts the chance to coat your stomach and satisfy your hunger.

### Sea Vegetables

Sea vegetables are generally classified according to color. They make great whole-food additions to your meals. Many people who advocate nutritional supplements encourage people to take something that contains whole foods—not just an individual vitamin that has been isolated from a food, but a product that will contain all the vitamins and minerals a food has to offer, even the ones that have not yet been discovered. Sea vegetables are a great natural way to get these important nutrients without consuming them through pill or powder form.

Sea vegetables include arame, hijiki, kombu, wakame, nori, and dulse, to name a few. They are an excellent source of protein, although not as good as the bean products. These can all be classified into one category and are allowed up to 4 ounces each day.

### Whole Cereal Grains

Whole cereal grains are generally classified as complex carbohydrates and they are included in that section as well. Those mentioned here are the highest in protein. Buckwheat (kasha), oats, and sorghum are included in the protein section. These grains are allowed up to a 1 cup cooked serving each day.

**Eggs**

Eggs are for the lacto-ovo vegetarian. They are allowable up to 6 each day. The type of fatty acid present in the egg is omega-3 fatty acid. Please don't consume the white of the egg without the egg yolk, because that's where the very healthy omega-3 is found. Organic eggs have more of the omega-3 fatty acid present, so keep this in mind if organic eggs are available where you live.

**Cheeses**

Again, this is for the lacto-ovo vegetarian.

> *Category 1:* hard or aged cheeses, including Swiss, muenster, cheddar, Brie, and any cheese not mentioned in category 2. They are allowed up to 3 ounces each day.
>
> *Category 2:* fresh or soft cheeses, such as cream cheese, pot cheese, farmer's cheese, cottage cheese, and ricotta. They are allowed up to 2 ounces each day.

## Complex Carbohydrates

**Vegetables**

> *Category 1:* salad vegetables, including all the different varieties of lettuces; and spinach, kale, fennel, mushrooms, olives, bok choy, celery, radishes, peppers, bean sprouts, and cucumbers. They are permitted up to 4 cups of lightly packed greens each day.
>
> *Category 2:* asparagus, green beans, broccoli, cauliflower, okra, eggplant, turnips, tomato, onion, leek, scallion, cabbage, avocado, snow pea pods, water chestnuts, zucchini, spaghetti squash, Brussels sprouts, artichoke hearts, collard greens, and dandelion greens. They are allowed up to 1 cup each day, cooked.
>
> *Category 3:* peas, beets, winter squashes, parsnips, and potatoes; and ethnic vegetables, including jicama, cassava, christophene, breadfruit, and plantains. These are not permitted.

**Grains**

These are the complex grains only and they include brown rice, wheat, rye, millet, and corn products. They must be complex—be sure to look for the word *whole* on food labels. These are allowable up to a ½-cup cooked serving twice each week, or 1 slice of whole-grain bread once each week.

## Desserts

The desserts available on this diet are those that appear in the recipe and menu section of this book. The only permissible commercially available dessert is sugar-free gelatin. This may be eaten in unlimited quantities, but be careful of the amount of aspartame you consume in a given day.

## Condiments

Please refer to chapter 8.

## Beverages

You must drink your body weight in kilograms, in ounces of water, each day. The water may be tap, filtered, spring, bottled, or carbonated.

Any beverage sweetened with sugar, including soda and fruit juice, is not permitted.

Diet soda is permitted up to 12 ounces each day. This includes any other artificially sweetened low-calorie beverage for a maximum total of 12 ounces each day.

### Alcohol

*Category 1:* scotch, bourbon, and other brown liquors. They are not permitted.

*Category 2:* gin, vodka, and other white liquors. They are not permitted.

*Category 3:* wine and beer are not permitted.

### Milk

*Category 1:* heavy cream is permitted up to 1 tablespoon per day. Yogurt (nonsweetened, unflavored) is allowed up to 4 ounces per week. Otherwise not permitted.

*Category 2:* unsweetened soy or rice milk is permitted up to 2 ounces three times per week.

## Fruit

*Category 1:* melons and berries. These are allowed up to ½ cup once each week.

*Category 2:* examples of these are grapefruits, plums, nectarines, and peaches. They are not permitted.

*Category 3:* examples of these are apples, kiwis, and oranges. They are not permitted.

*Category 4:* tropical fruits, such as bananas, mangoes, papaya, guava, and pineapple. They are not permitted.

As you can see, it is entirely possible to enjoy the health benefits of a higher-protein diet while still remaining a vegetarian. It just takes a manipulation of the currently accepted vegetarian diet, which in my opinion is unhealthy, and replacing some of the pasta or bread choices with nonanimal sources of protein. This version of Thin For Good will not only trim your waistline, but it will also open you up to an entire world of foods that you may not be aware exists.

There is one warning: *Do not combine the two diets, vegetarian and non-vegetarian.* I do not offer the vegetarian diet as an option for the majority of readers. I offer it so those who are vegetarians can be healthier ones, and lose weight, too.

And remember, you vegetarians should not forget to include the mind-body medicines that are so vital to my diet program. Their use is not optional, and I encourage you to try to find meditations of your own that have significant meaning in your own life.

## THE ELEVEN EMOTIONAL LEVELS OF EATING
# LEVEL 11: CONTENTMENT

At last!—the final emotional level I see people go through in their quest for thinness. Not everyone will reach this stage, partly because it is the scariest emotional level. This means that you must be happy enough and have enough self-involvement to be able to make a commitment to the new you. You have to be content with whatever shape the new you may take—whether it be the 50 pounds lighter you wanted to be or just the 35 pounds lighter you have been able to achieve right now.

We have to become more accepting of ourselves and where we are in our lives. This is the only way we will ever be able to have the commitment we need. We have to accept that dieting will be a way of life for us for the rest of our lives. Yes, the forever phase may not be as strict as the initiation phase, but there will always be some level of dieting going on in our lives. We have to be as content with that knowledge as we are with our new bodies.

It is harder to be content than you would think. Most of us have never led our lives feeling content. We are much more used to feeling miserable or discontented, and for these emotions we know how to act. This is our opportunity to learn how to be content. Not an easy task, but rewarding in the long run. Please answer the following questions to help you explore some of the issues you may have with contentment:

1. What makes me feel contented?
2. Do I ever feel contented?
3. Who makes me feel content just to be around?
4. What do I accept no matter what?
5. Whom do I accept no matter what?

### Bonus Questions: What do I accept about myself? What don't I accept about myself?

This is the key to being content. If you can answer these questions, especially the bonus round, you will have a pretty good understanding about your level of contentment. We have to be content even with the things we do not accept about ourselves; otherwise those things may hurt us. We need to learn how to be content with our new and possibly improved selves, no matter who that might be. If we can master that task, we are well on our way to being able to live our lives with the improvements we have just made.

**Mind-Body Medicines to Learn about Contentment:**

- The seed you plant is the fruit you don't eat.

- You must desire the end result of being thinner and healthier more than immediate gratification.
- Thinness must be created.

**Recipes That May Help with Contentment:**
- Nutty Grain
- Strawberries with Almond Custard

You have now been presented with my eleven emotional levels of eating. I don't think there is a reader of this book who has never eaten emotionally at some point in her or his life. I hope these levels will teach you why you eat in certain ways and therefore provide you with the tools you will need to overcome the cycle of emotional eating. I would like you to use what I have said about the emotional levels combined with the medicines for your mind to make a positive impact on your weight and your health. You may use these over and over again as you see fit. You may also choose not to use certain ones that may not apply to you. Whatever the case, you can be sure they will play a strong role in how well you succeed in this program.

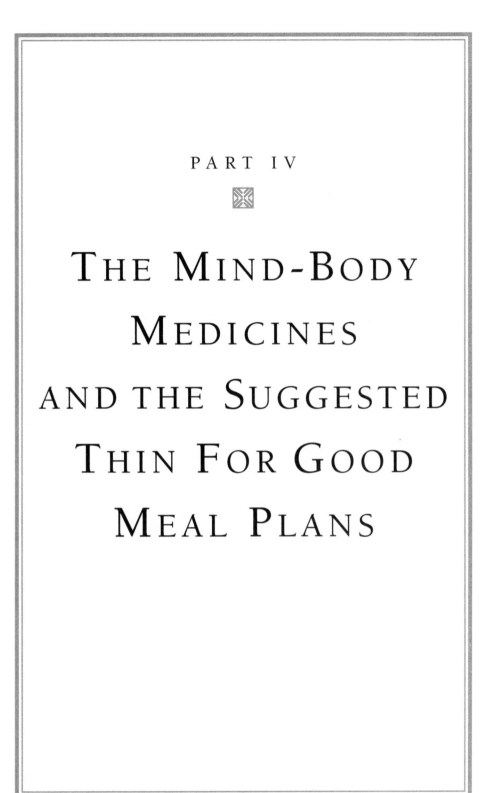

# THE MIND-BODY MEDICINES AND THE SUGGESTED THIN FOR GOOD MEAL PLANS

# CHAPTER 12

# Mind Over Calories

Mind Over Calories is the concept that has enabled me to keep my weight off successfully. It is a series of credos, developed over the past decade, that I live with daily that help me live life as a thinner person. Now I am happy to be able to share it with a much larger audience than just my patients.

I call these credos my mind-body medicines, and there will be one to help you get through each of the first thirty days of this new diet plan.

The key to Mind Over Calories is the simple concept that losing weight and keeping weight off are easier to accomplish—and certainly most successful—when we take time to do some psychological work. In order to never put excess weight on again, your mind must play an important role in the process; and in order to get that weight off in the first place, you must learn new ways of dealing with food.

Mind Over Calories is a concept I came across accidentally in my multi-decade battle with weight issues. Once I had lost the weight that I had wanted, I was faced with the age-old question of "now what?" Since I had no support from my family, and I learned how to lose weight all on my own, I now needed to learn how to stay that way while being surrounded by overweight people who looked at me as if I was the one with the problem, not them.

## Thin People Don't Worry

It's my guess that naturally thin people never know what we overweight people go through when it comes to food. Those of us who do have a weight problem constantly worry if we are eating too much fat, too much sugar, too much cholesterol, too much carbohydrate, too much anything. And then we worry that something is going to happen to us as a result of our eating habits—heart disease, cancer, stroke. If it is not one thing, it will surely be another. There is always something overweight, or now formerly overweight, people worry about when it comes to food.

The mind-body advice in this book is the manual for revealing the mysteries of your mind as it relates to food. I have already given you the weight loss tools in the previous chapters. Now you need to combine the two sets of instructions into the most powerful weight loss program that you have ever experienced.

Mind Over Calories is similar to a Buddhist concept. When you stop wanting something, that's precisely when you'll get it. Stopping the desire is the key, and believe me, this is harder to do than just saying you are going to do it.

That was my epiphany, and that is how I have been living most of my life—trying to rid myself of the desire. It has been at the times in my life when I start worrying about what I am eating that I start to gain weight again. During the past years, I have refined this concept, primarily through the study and exploration of various spiritual concepts and ideas. As you read through these next few chapters you may find many of the concepts that I present familiar, because I have simply combined the best concepts from everything I have studied and have applied them to food and dieting.

This chapter and the ones that follow are as important to the success of my diet as any others that have come before. In fact, they may be even more important, because if you can master the ideas proposed in these chapters, then you have a tremendous chance of successfully losing weight and keeping it off for the rest of your life.

Success is measured not by whether or not you can lose weight, but by whether or not you can remain thin over the course of a lifetime. Your mind holds the key to true long-term success. The next chapter is going to give you the first thirty days of your new nutritional lifestyle program. It is going to include a suggested menu for each day and a daily dose of mind-body medicine. That is what you need in order to be successful.

I live my life by these rules, and I have been a successful thin person for over half my life. I can now say that I have been thin longer than I was ever overweight. I am going to share many of my thoughts with you about how I have managed to accomplish that goal, and how I have managed to help patients do the same thing.

## Feed Your Mind

For the first thirty days of the diet, there will be a different dose of mind-body medicine for every day of the week. After that, you may repeat those that work best for you, as not all of these doses will have the same meaning for everyone who uses them. So if you come across one that has no meaning at all to you, try to alter it in some way so that it does. Remember, these doses are not set in stone, and if you come across more suitable ones, I would love to hear from you, so I may include them in my next book.

Feel free to use whichever ones you want to use, whenever you want to use them. They should become your saying for the day. I want you to refer to this dose constantly during the day, whenever you feel an urge to do something you shouldn't be doing, and at any time of the day when you feel you need some inspiration. We all need inspiration and these 30 daily doses have changed my life and the lives of many of my patients. I encourage you to use them and take full advantage of the power they hold. I encourage you to write them on cards and keep them with you so you can refer to them. Make multiple index cards and keep a set in your purse, jacket pocket, on the refrigerator, in your office, or wherever you will be on that particular day.

There is no right or wrong way to feel when reading these words of inspiration. If you don't feel anything from the first one, then move on to the next, or try to see what the potential benefit may be even if you don't get it right away.

All I ask is that you read all of them, read my explanation of them, then take a couple of minutes to see how they can make an impact in your life.

This program will work for you if you give the mind-body medicines a chance. In all my years of practicing nutritional medicine, these daily doses have been the key to my patients' losing weight and keeping it off.

The doses are meant to be used to inspire you, and never as an excuse to go off the diet. The diet can be successful even without these inspirational sayings—but I find it more successful with them.

CHAPTER 13

✕

# The Mind-Body Medicines and Meal Plans—Week 1

## A Word on the Menus

These are just sample menus for the first thirty days of your new nutritional lifestyle program. They may be used for any stage, male or female. They are not set in stone, so you should not feel as if this is what you must eat to stay with the Thin For Good program. Always refer to chapter 8 for the overall guidelines, and to chapters 9 or 10 for full details. I encourage you to be creative.

These menus, and the recipes in Part VII, should give you some idea of how creative you can be with the foods I have listed as permissible—depending, of course, on which stage of the diet you are in. These menus are those I give to my patients after I have gone over their blood work with them. It is quite easy to devise menus from all the choices that are available to you.

Having created them, I can attest that not only do they produce meals that are good tasting, but they are also fun to make!

As for what to drink, I always recommend you drink water or flavored seltzer, which is why liquids are not included in the menu section. Please refer to the necessary chapter that corresponds to your stage and sex for any particulars.

A note: In the recipe section, you will notice that I included two additional salad dressings: Lemon-Dill and Simple French Vinaigrette. These may be substituted for any of the other dressings listed in the menu section.

I encourage you to create your own recipes, and if they work out, I'd love you to share them with me—perhaps I will include them in my next book. There is always room to learn from my patients and friends, and some of the recipes that follow are from patients and readers of my last book. I hope you enjoy them as much as I did compiling them. Happy eating!

My daily doses for the mind will help you get through the diet and thereby make your weight loss a lifelong success story. Essentially, these are "arguments" or reasons why you should remain on your diet or on the maintenance part of the diet. There is one for each of the first thirty days of your new program. After that, you may simply start over again from the beginning or simply reuse the ones you found the most valuable. To make it even easier, chapter 21 contains more mind-body medicines you may find useful.

Week 1 is a relatively easy week to get through because you will be really motivated at this point in the diet. You are ready for what it takes to lose that weight or get healthy. I use this week to teach the basics of the mind-set that will help you to be a successful dieter. Please keep in mind that there is a recipe for every dish I have listed in these menu suggestions in Part VII.

# Day 1

## Menu Suggestions

| | |
|---|---|
| Breakfast: | Baked Eggs |
| Lunch: | Heart-Art |
| Dinner: | Asparagus and Sesame Chicken Soup |
| | Oriental Shrimp and Broccoli Stir-Fry |

### DAILY DOSE:
### Remember the power of Mind Over Calories.

You must take control over what goes on in your mind, at least as it relates to food. It's far better for you if you are not so obsessed with everything that goes into your mouth. If you make your food choices from the proper foods, this ceases to be a problem, even if you have a few indulgences along the way, such as occasionally eating foods that are not actually on the diet.

# Day 2

## Menu Suggestions

| | |
|---|---|
| Breakfast: | Shrimp Omelet |
| Lunch: | Luciano |
| Dinner: | White Gazpacho |
| | Roasted Fish |

### DAILY DOSE:
### Make a commitment to being thinner.

This sounds easy, but it's not. And yet this is a very big concept. It must be understood in its entirety, because it can have a big impact on how successful you can be with your new diet. Changing your diet is truly about making a commitment—a very serious commitment, one that should be as serious as a marriage (maybe even more so, these days), or as serious as your job.

I'm not just talking about lip service. Remaining on this diet, or any diet for that matter, must become one of the primary driving forces of your life. Let's say that you've made a commitment to dieting, to being thinner, or just to being healthy. If you truly make a commitment, you will do everything in your power to honor that commitment and, as a result, your new diet will work. If you have the proper commitment, there is simply no other choice. You will do whatever it takes to reach the goal. By having a commitment to this new nutritional lifestyle program, every action you take, every food you consider eating, every time you decide to exercise, every time you decide not to exercise, gets you closer to or farther from your goal.

We are all goal-oriented individuals, but let's be honest, we never let that goal-driven behavior influence our food choices. Food is one of the few areas in our lives where we allow something to control us, rather than the other way around. We are lenient. We all have those easy excuses readily available: "I had a bad day," or "I'm not feeling well," or "I had a fight with my husband/wife." Frankly, it doesn't matter what the excuse is because I've heard them all. That's all they are—excuses to give ourselves license to indulge, which only takes us farther from our original goal of losing weight and getting healthy. If you are truly committed to being thin or getting healthy, you will be able to make the right decisions when it comes to food.

Make a commitment to the future. It is important to know what you want the future to look like. Do you want to be overweight, or do you want to be thinner and healthier? You must have this clear picture in your mind. If you can do this, and you know what the future should look like, then you can go about doing the things it takes to reach that goal and create the future you desire.

You may feel that there is no way we can ever know what the future holds. Think about it. You had an idea about what you wanted to be when you grew up. Therefore, you did what it took to get you there. For instance, I knew I wanted to be a physician from an early age. So I had to go to college and medical school and scores of other things had to happen before I actually fulfilled my dream of becoming a doctor. Careers obviously take a high priority in our life, but the same commitment to a very reachable goal has to be securely in place in order for a diet to be successful. Why should careers take all of our focus, when our health is far more important?

If you want to be thinner and healthier, and are truly committed to this goal, then that chocolate cake, birthday party, dinner with friends becomes not an obstacle, but an opportunity to showcase your commitment to the new you. The commitment takes precedence and it becomes easy to make the right decision. That's not to say that you will always make the right decision, or that there won't be detours along the way. *All you need to do is to keep the end point in sight and make that commitment.* The rest should be easy.

# Day 3

## Menu Suggestions

Breakfast:   Corned Beef Hash
Lunch:       Cold Sesame Chicken Salad
Dinner:      Ham Steak
             Cucumber Sauté

### DAILY DOSE:
### *Realize the power of your thoughts and talking about dieting.*

This is a concept that has helped me keep my commitment to being thinner and healthier. Simply put, you must truly mean what you say and think. Also, you must realize that what you say and do has an impact on those around you. If you truly act and speak like a dieter, that is how people will treat you. They will give you room to diet. There will be no coercion, no bending of the arm, and no temptations offered from those around you if you simply are true to what you say. You can only be treated as you expect to be treated.

We all think we mean what we say, but how many times have you said something you didn't really mean? We say things all day long that we don't mean, and this has a direct influence on the way we diet; when we say we are on a diet, it's too easy for that to become one of the many things that we don't mean. You must know that in your words and thoughts there is the power to do what you want to do in your lifetime, whether it be personal or professional.

I have treated many executives and celebrities who have a problem in realizing how this simple concept applies to their diets. Ironically, these people would never have gotten to where they are today without having a high level of commitment or without knowing the power of what they say in their professional lives. Yet, when it comes to what they eat, they have a definite problem, one that I think most of us share. We don't place enough emphasis on the power we have over the food we put in our mouths. We are the ones eating it, and we are the ones who can make the correct decisions by realizing and giving power to our thoughts and words.

Repeat after me: *I am going to lose weight. I am going to stay on my diet. I am going to win this battle and get healthy.* If you allow those words and thoughts to have significance and power, you will never be able to do anything that will jeopardize your necessary path to thinness.

# Day 4

## Menu Suggestions

Breakfast: Cowboy Roll-Up
Lunch:     Chicken Licken
Dinner:    Baby Bok Choy
           Beef Stroganoff

### DAILY DOSE:
### *Expectations about weight loss outcomes affect results.*

Whenever we enter into something, no matter what it is—a new job, a new relationship, a new diet—we have an expectation of what is going to happen. And that expectation is generally met, whether it's good or bad. Unfortunately, because of all the baggage we carry around, the expectation is often a negative. I encourage you to go into this diet without any preconceived notions that you have made yourself or that you may have heard from others about what this diet is going to do for you. I encourage you to undertake this new nutritional lifestyle plan as if you are seeing a low-carb diet for the first time.

I honestly feel that this plan is a novel concept. I can guarantee that you have never been on a program that took into account your sex and stage of life and gave you a mind-body program to lose weight. You should enter into this program with no expectations whatsoever.

Subconsciously, our expectations influence the outcome of anything we try to achieve. You must try to avoid this at all costs when you are on this diet. I want you to embark on this diet not knowing what is going to happen, because whatever is going to happen is the right thing.

Sure, we all go on a diet expecting to lose weight. That is only human, and a natural response. I have had many patients come to me only because they wanted to lose weight. After examining them, I found them to have high cholesterol, high blood pressure, diabetes type II, or some other incidental, yet important, condition that they didn't even know they had. After the first six weeks, I will usually repeat a patient's blood work, more to reassure the patient than because I am concerned with the results—because I know they will be better than when the patient initially presented.

I then review the new blood work with the patient. Let's say her cholesterol has dropped 50 points, or her triglyceride level has dropped 100 points, or her blood pressure is within the normal range when before it wasn't, or her blood sugar is markedly improved. Yet she hasn't lost any weight. And do you know what she cares the most about? Of course, it's the weight. She often will not care that she has never felt better in her life, or that a serious medical problem has been corrected.

This is often the patient's first excuse to stop the diet, even though the diet might be the right thing. It is usually the first step toward setting yourself up to feel like a failure when you are not a failure at all. In this particular situation, the person has practically given herself another five years of life, yet she feels as if she has failed. I think this still goes back to the concept that knowing how to be a failure is easier than knowing how to be a winner.

We are more comfortable failing. Don't be. You can't allow that negative feeling to corrupt the dieting process. Know that there is going to be a little discomfort in this dieting process and accept the fact. Accept the good things that happen as easily as you accept the bad things.

Let's discuss the whole concept of "not losing enough." What is that all about? What is not enough? Not enough for whom? Are we in a race? And if so, whom are we racing against? These are negative thoughts when it comes to dieting. These are excuses you are setting up in your own mind, so when you make a decision to participate in a behavior that will not lead you to your goal, you'll think it's okay because "this diet wasn't working for me anyway."

Stop using excuses. Have no expectations about results that can jeopardize the outcome. *Know something good is going to happen and go with that.* Be happy with whatever good thing comes out of your experience with this new diet. Don't jeopardize the good results you see because the outcome isn't everything you might expect it to be. It will be what it will be.

# Day 5

## Menu Suggestions

Breakfast:  Traditional Omelet
Lunch:      Burger a la Caesar
Dinner:     Avocado Soup
            Sautéed Filet of Sole with Vegetables

### DAILY DOSE:
### *Energy has no limitations in our drive for thinness.*

There is no limit to what you can achieve if you can tap into your significant inner energy and the even more endless energy of the universe. If you are a religious person, you can think of this energy in terms of God or whichever spiritual being you worship.

Most of us believe there is some universal energy available to us that we can tap into, no matter what we call it. This driving force, which can also help us with dieting, has no limitations on what it can attain and create. We set up those limitations. We create the barriers. They are not built in. We must learn to un-create these limitations by realizing the boundless energy that is available to us, if we allow it to be.

Create a thinner you. Create a healthier you. This can be accomplished if you believe it can. By knowing it can happen, things can change. All you have to do is realize the possibility that other things exist. Know it. Know things can change. If Edison had never conceived that there could be a light bulb, we'd all still be in the dark. Science uses this concept to expand our horizons on a daily basis. Why shouldn't you?

We need to know that there does not have to be any limitation to what we can achieve if we want it badly enough. If you have been overweight your whole life, you should know you can still change that. Being overweight the first thirty or forty or even fifty years of your life does not force you to be overweight for the remaining years. All it means is that you were overweight for those years. That's it. Now you can move on.

Don't assign those overweight years any more meaning than what they are: simply put, it was the way you were then, or even the way you are now. Those heavyweight years do not mean you are a failure now. Those years of excess weight do not mean you were meant to be heavy your whole life. They do not mean that you were never meant to shop in the regular department of your favorite store. They do not mean you are destined to have your first heart attack at age forty-five, like your father did. All it means is that you were once overweight or once unhealthy. Do not assign it any more meaning than it has.

*Now, create a new story from the endless possibilities of the energy, and make it a thinner version of the story.*

# Day 6

## Menu Suggestions

Breakfast:  Ham and Eggs
Lunch:      Top-Hat Burger
Dinner:     Cauliflower Latkes
            Chicken and Sausage Bundles

### DAILY DOSE:
### *Our body creates a desire for the things we shouldn't have, especially when dieting.*

I use this thought to help myself and my patients deal with food cravings, something you may be experiencing right about now. Do you ever get cravings that are almost out of control for certain foods, especially when you are dieting? It happens to all of us. It is important to know that it is a universal phenomenon and that you are not the only person this happens to. Food cravings can make us irritable, frustrated, and generally unpleasant to be around. This is the daily dose that is going to help you to overcome those peaks and valleys. My diet will help you physically control these feelings. Once the mind and the body are combined, the negativity can be released and you no longer have to hold on to it as a form of expression. What this then creates is the need for something to fill its place. Nature abhors a vacuum, so you can use this mind-body medicine to create something new, a new place to hang your old hat.

The thing that separates successful dieters from the ones who will fall back into their old habits is knowing that it is your mind that is creating the desire for the food that you shouldn't have. There is no other basis for the craving, especially with this diet because it regulates your blood sugar so well that you should never have any cravings, at least physiologically.

I have found that by simply recognizing that the desire is coming from a negative energy place, it is much easier to resist temptation. I introduce the concept of negative energy here for a reason. I believe that just as there is a lot of positive, creative energy in the world, there is negative energy as well. Our desire for the wrong things, for things that are bad for us, comes from this negative energy. We often don't see this energy as negative, especially when it comes to food, because, after all, how important is it really to stay away from that piece of chocolate? But if you are committed to being thin or being healthy, then it is just as important to stay away from that piece of chocolate as it is, for instance, not to break the law.

We use negative energy to build up such resistance to the things that are good for us that it may take a tremendous amount of work to lose weight. So many layers of resistance build up over the years that it is no wonder that it is easy to lose the weight but so difficult to keep it off. In the end, we make it much more difficult than it ever has to be. Have you ever worked yourself up into a frenzy over something, like visiting your in-laws, only to have the event take place without a hitch? It's the same principle.

Let me give you another example. On one level there may be a thought, however subconscious, that you should never look good, because of your desire to remain unattractive or to go through life unnoticed, or whatever the reason might be. I'd bet there are many reasons that all contribute to why we are overweight. The layers run deep and many of them may never be resolved. But you can learn to live with them and still be a successful dieter. I'd like you to take a moment and deeply explore some of the reasons why you may be overweight and write them down here:

1. _____

2. _____

3. _____

4. _____

*Just know that the desire to do badly on a diet is in all of us. Know it, accept it, and move on. Make the commitment, acknowledge the negative energy behind the desire, and ignore the craving.*

# Day 7

## Menu Suggestions

Breakfast:  Sunday Special Treat
Lunch:      Taxco Topper
Dinner:     Springtime Spaghetti Squash
            Beefsteaks with Gorgonzola Sauce

### DAILY DOSE:
### *Don't let what is happening to you control*
### *how well you do on your diet.*

This dose is one of my favorites and maybe that's because it helps me the most. Do you admit to sometimes eating for a reason other than hunger? Would you say that you are an emotional eater? Do you get moody if you don't eat? I would answer yes to each of those questions.

We must keep in mind that eating should occur only when we are hungry and not for any other reason. We should not be eating when we are sad, happy, upset, self-destructive, because the food is there and you don't want to see it go to waste, because you simply want to be polite, or because you can't say no. The list goes on and on, and I'm sure that you could list a few of your own excuses that you've used from time to time to help you justify in your mind the eating mistakes you've made along the way. Write some of those down in the spaces provided so that you know some of the things you are going to need to overcome in order to be the success you want to be:

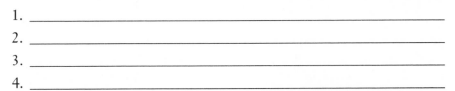

1. _____
2. _____
3. _____
4. _____

Just because you had a bad day at work, or because you broke up with your boyfriend, or because you had a fight with your wife and she was the one who wanted you to go on this diet in the first place, or any one of a million other circumstances that may affect your life does not mean that you should go off your diet and indulge to make yourself feel better. Rationalizations, such as, "It's just this once" or "I deserve this" just don't cut it.

None of these excuses fly if you truly are committed to losing weight. There are always going to be circumstances that arise in our lives, unless we become hermits (and I'm sure even then some of us would find an excuse to blame something or someone other than ourselves for our bad eating behaviors) when we are going to have the urge to turn to food. Food is comforting, food will make me feel better—NOT! I can't tell you how many times I have heard patients say, myself included, how much worse they felt after the indulgence, how they will never do that again because they felt so bad. The good feeling you experience from that food will probably be only a momentary thing. Don't let it ruin your diet. Step back from the situation. Take a deep breath. Leave the room if you need to, and spend a couple of minutes in what I call "quiet time." I would bet your desire to eat for the wrong reason will disappear if you don't give in to it.

Don't let circumstances control you. You are in control over what goes into your mouth at all times. Take back control of your life in the matter of food, even if you have no control over some of the other things that may be going on in your life. *Use food as your control mechanism rather than one more aspect of your life over which you have no control.*

※

# CHAPTER 14

# The Mind-Body Medicines and Meal Plans—Week 2

You've gotten through the first week. Congratulations. That's a big accomplishment because it's probably the second hardest week of your diet. The first week is never the hardest, because in my experience people are at their most motivated during the first week and therefore willing to make the most sacrifices. I find that it is about the third week that people have the most difficulty. If you can maintain your diet until then and then get over that hump, things will get easier as you get programmed and acclimated to your new and improved way of eating.

## Day 8

### Menu Suggestions

Breakfast: Shrimp Surprise Roll-Up
Lunch: Cyndi
Dinner: Oriental Shrimp
Easy Pilaf
Chicken Sautéed with Raspberry Vinegar

DAILY DOSE:
*The person who works the hardest at his or her diet appreciates the most.*

At first glance, this concept is fairly self-explanatory. Simply put, if you truly do the work involved in this diet, you are going to appreciate the results. That's one way of looking at this statement. The other, more powerful way of looking at it is: you should never judge yourself against others because you never know what other people had to do to get the results they did.

You can't compare yourself to the next person. Dieting is an individual thing, and anyone who says it isn't is wrong. Don't compare yourself to your husband or your girlfriend or your sister. It is an impossible and ultimately self-defeating habit, just another excuse in the long line of excuses that we build into our repertoire of dieting problems. The only comparison you should make is to yourself.

It is important that you not only appreciate the results, but also the hard work that went into attaining those results. It can't and should not be a constant battle. Just because something is a struggle doesn't mean that it has to be hard work. The difficulty level is one being superimposed from the outside. If it is your thoughts and your own actions that are making the diet difficult, that's where the trouble lies. The hardest work should not be your mental state but rather doing the exercise, and making drastic changes in your perception of food, in what food means to you, and in the role it plays in your life. This is an opportune moment to think yourself thin. Only you are standing in your way—no one and nothing else.

By making the tough choices—to not join your friends for dinner at the pasta restaurant, to not go to that party, or to not have that piece of cake that is just sitting in the freezer calling out your name—you are going to appreciate the rewards in the long term.

*Make the hard part of this diet the actual work you have to do, not all the mind games we can all force ourselves to go through when we are doing something we really don't want to do even though it is the best thing for us.*

# Day 9

## *Menu Suggestions*

Breakfast: Nordic Omelet
Lunch:     Feta and Beef Salad
Dinner:    Bibb Lettuce with Fresh Herb Dressing
           Monk Kabobs
Dessert:   Ace's Strawberries with Almond Custard

### DAILY DOSE:
*Take full responsibility for being overweight.*

For the most part, it is our fault we are overweight. Yes, there are some medical conditions that predispose us to being overweight, but what I speak of here is our almost innate way of telling ourselves that there are all these outside influences that cause our weight issues.

We've heard them all before, and many of us have said them ourselves. "Oh, I have a slow metabolism" or "I had to taste the dessert in order to be polite." There are a million of these excuses and I want you to stop using them right now. You must accept responsibility for your weight problem. If you don't have a weight problem and are doing this diet for health reasons, then you must accept full responsibility for your own health. For the most part, we are the ones who overindulged, thought the ice cream was more important than our waistlines, or worse, didn't appreciate the outcome that our behavior would have.

Think of your pet or your children or your job—things for which you have complete responsibility. You would never not feed your pet, not know where your children are and what they are doing (at least to the best of your ability), or not report to your boss on your progress. Yet we almost never apply those same rigid principles to our dieting. Many of our common everyday responsibilities become second nature to us. Making the proper food decisions can be another one of those simple, second-nature responses if you let it become that easy. Fight the negative impulses to do the wrong thing. Don't fight the positive impulses to do the right thing. Allow changes in your habits to take place. It is only human to resist change. This is one area in your life where you must fight that. In this situation, change is good.

Remember, you were the one who ate all the food; no one forced you. You were the one who either cooked it, ordered it in, ate it in a restaurant, or had someone make it for you. If you can do that, then you can make the necessary changes so that the food you do eat is the food that can help you to be healthy and lose weight.

*Take back the responsibility. You can handle one more thing you are responsible for. Follow the rules of the diet. Act as if your life depends on it, because it probably does.*

# Day 10

## *Menu Suggestions*

    Breakfast:  Sunday on a Wednesday Eggs
    Lunch:      South-of-the-Border Burger
    Dinner:     Gen's Green Beans
                Roman Turkey Cutlets

### DAILY DOSE:
### *Take full responsibility for cheating.*

I like to throw this one in on the tenth day of the diet, because I have found that this is when people begin to see results and they sometimes convince themselves to cheat because they've been so good. Taking responsibility for this cheating may be one of the simplest concepts to understand if you understand the Day 9 concept.

You are the one responsible for the cheating you do. No one else. For dieters, cheating is unacceptable.

If you are using these mind-body medicines for the maintenance portion of the diet, cheating is probably something that you are going to do at one time or another. We are only human and we find it difficult to change our inherent nature to do the wrong things.

Many of us make excuse after excuse about why we have eaten the wrong foods. I had to because . . . —you can fill in the blank here. No one forced you to eat anything. No one made you do anything. Since most of us are adults, we would almost never think of succumbing to peer pressure at this point in our lives, yet that is exactly what we do when we make the wrong food choices.

Remember, you are the one totally and completely responsible for what goes into your mouth. Make that a powerful statement and use its power. Remember the power you have in your thoughts and actions. Don't be afraid of this statement, thereby allowing it to destroy the good work you've accomplished in the past nine days.

If you take responsibility for the cheating, and are truly committed to this new lifestyle program, you may find it impossible to cheat. The commitment makes it impossible to do anything that is not on the diet. The responsibility is all yours. You don't fool anyone but yourself when you cheat. Many of my patients have admitted to me that they are only harming their own chances at thinness and health, not mine, by lying to me or, at the very least, stretching the truth.

If you do find yourself cheating, and I don't advocate this position, then take the responsibility for the cheat and move on. It was only a cheat. Period, end of story. Don't make it into something else and don't use it as your excuse to go off the diet. Immediately get back on the diet. Don't wait another meal, or another day. You cheated once and yes, it was cheating, but now just begin again, immediately.

*Use this tenth day to know that everything you do in terms of making food choices is your direct responsibility. You have the power to make the proper decisions, so do it.*

# Day 11

## Menu Suggestions

Breakfast:  California Roll-Up
Lunch:      The Temptation
Dinner:     Romaine Lettuce with Gorgonzola Dressing
            Swordfish

## DAILY DOSE:
### Work to change the negative dieting situation.

Have you ever been in a situation where it feels as if something is happening to you, yet you seem to have no responsibility for what's going on and the outcome is anyone's guess? I'm sure that has happened to most of you, because I know it has happened to me, especially when I am trying to lose weight. When a craving hits, it's almost as if I have no control. Once I let go of the control, the floodgates open and all food is open and fair game. It's a scary situation.

I've used this daily dose to help me out of that downward spiral, and the concept is really quite simple: *We have to work at dieting.* Dieting must become our job, our life's work, our motivation. I have found that many overweight people, myself once included, think dieting is just following a set of rules that may or may not be complicated, and then the weight will just fall off. That sometimes happens, and that's a good thing. But, believe me, the majority of the time and for the majority of people it just doesn't happen that easily. Even if it does, you still have to deal with the problem of keeping the weight off. So, if you are one of the lucky ones who can lose weight on almost any diet, consider that you wouldn't be reading this book if you were truly a successful dieter before. Use this mind-body medicine to help you break the cycle and the frustration of yo-yo dieting.

Whether the initial weight loss is fast or slow, you still have to make changes in your lifestyle. And if you want to succeed forever, these changes are going to have to become more or less permanent. Admittedly, this takes work. This is not something that is going to happen overnight or even within these first thirty days of the diet. It is a lifelong commitment and a lifelong battle, even if you lose the weight and manage to be very good at keeping it off.

I should know, because I was overweight and now I live my life as a much lighter person. This takes work, a tremendous amount of work. I constantly mind what I eat. I exercise often. I often turn down food I would love to have. I often turn down dinner party invitations if I know I will be unable to eat the food that will be served. It is all worth it to me, because I love the end result of all this work. Believe me, it ain't easy. But by this time I'm sure I'm not telling you anything you don't already know.

Use this mind-body medicine to let yourself know that a diet takes work, not only in the beginning when things are relatively easy, but for your whole life. I have to work at dieting every day, and so will you. Dieting must become just another one of those things that we do on an almost everyday basis and hope it becomes almost a subconscious effort. There is no room for any of the negative energies we constantly ascribe to the dieting process.

*Dieting has no beginning and no end.* It just is. I know that if you keep this in mind, the bigger picture can become clearer. For me, and for many of my patients, it makes it that much easier not to do the wrong thing.

# Day 12

## Menu Suggestions

Breakfast:  Mushroom, Ham, and Brie Omelet
Lunch:      Prince
Dinner:     Bacon-Wrapped Scallops
            Greek Quinoa
            Grilled Boneless Leg of Lamb

### DAILY DOSE:
### *Stop building walls against losing weight.*

Have you set up barriers to dieting? If you answered "not me," then I think you're fooling yourself. At one point or another, all of us have done this, whether subconsciously or downright blatantly. We attack one barrier only to find another pop up to take its place almost simultaneously. When we set up these barriers over and over again, we set ourselves up repeatedly for failure. Essentially, we are dooming ourselves to a lifetime of unhealthy behaviors simply because we can't get out from behind our walls.

Many of us have built so many walls or barriers that are so ingrained in our psyches and have become so much a part of who we are that we can't even name some of them.

Is it your mother who upsets you and makes you want to eat? Is it your mother who wants to feed you all the time, as was the case with me? Is it your fear of being attractive that is your undoing? Is it just too many social gatherings your ego can't say no to? Is it because the food is in the house and you can't see it go to waste? Is it simply your lack of willpower?

Is it the frustration of having to learn a whole new set of dieting rules? Is it to frustrate your husband? Is it denial that you won't ever get a heart attack just like your father/brother/best friend did?

There are hundreds of these excuses, and before you read any further I want you to write down a few of the ones that you have used in the past:

1. _____
2. _____
3. _____
4. _____

Whether you can relate to the examples I gave or not, I'm sure you have issues of your own. But whatever they are, they all come down to the same thing—an obstacle that prevents you from achieving the goal you think you want.

You need to understand that the more barriers there are, the more difficult it is to get through them. A new barrier forms every time you try a new diet and fail. These barriers start to build on themselves, and each one fortifies the one that has come before. The more you allow those layers to build up and fail to do any work to help remove them, the more difficult it will be to be a successful dieter. This is not to say that you won't be able to lose weight on this diet if you follow the rules and do nothing else. But I want more than that for you. I want you to be successful in the long run and make this the last diet book you ever buy. Unless you realize what harm you may be doing by building these barriers, you'll never overcome them. Stop another one from forming and do this diet right the first time. *Realize the barrier, and overcome it. If you don't even recognize that something is a barrier, it makes it that much more difficult to get around.*

# Day 13

## Menu Suggestions

| | |
|---|---|
| Breakfast: | Spinach Pie |
| Lunch: | Saltimbocca |
| Dinner: | Spinach and Ricotta Dumplings |
| | Korean Short Ribs |
| Dessert: | Lemon Cheesecake Square |

### DAILY DOSE:
### *The seed you plant is the fruit you don't eat.*

I changed this saying because I don't allow early phase dieters to have too much fruit. The fruit issue is not as important as the heart of the concept. It's another very simple thought: If you plant oranges you get oranges; you will never get cucumbers.

When it comes to dieting, you cannot expect the outcome to be good if you eat the wrong foods. If you eat that brownie, the ice cream, or whatever the indulgence is, how can you possibly think it won't change the outcome you are trying to achieve?

You might wonder, "What happens if I cheat just a little?" or "How bad can two glasses of wine with dinner be?" It can be very bad—destructive in fact. It all depends on which phase of my diet you are on, and whether or not you think alcohol should be an important part of your life. Cheating just a little is like cheating just a lot. If you cheat, that is the seed you plant. You are never going to get thin that way. It just won't happen.

Please keep in mind that for the most part, your diets are going to affect you over the course of your lifetime. It is not something that is going to have an immediate effect except in cases of diabetes. There is a bigger picture to keep in mind here. Don't let a momentary indulgence cost you a lifetime of good health, because indulgences are cumulative—they add up.

Remember, it takes a long time to grow a plant from a seed. We are not looking for immediate effects—okay, some of us are, but we shouldn't be. Instead, we are looking for a lifetime of positive health benefits. What you put into this diet is what you will get out of it. When you are using this concept for dieting, just remember that what you put in your mouth—and I mean every last bit of it—is going to affect the bottom line (or the waistline); for maintenance dieters, look at the bigger picture before making those indulgences. After all, *you truly are what you eat.*

# Day 14

## Menu Suggestions

Breakfast:  Louisville Oeufs!
Lunch:      Salad Nicoise
Dinner:     Zucchini Spears
            Senoran Steaks

### DAILY DOSE:
*You must desire the end result of being thinner and healthier more than immediate gratification.*

This is really an easy concept to understand, yet it is a more difficult one to put into practice. Most of us have spent the better part of our lives in pursuit of immediate gratification. The baby boomer generation practically epitomizes the concept.

The pursuit of immediate gratification is perfect for people who like food, and ultimately this pursuit will be one of your downfalls. If you didn't like food, you probably would not be reading a book on the subject of nutrition. Most of us are fortunate enough to be able to get food whenever we want it, usually in the form that we want it. Some corporations have built empires around providing us with food we know and recognize instantly no matter where we are on the planet.

I believe this need for instant food began when we were infants. Whenever we started to cry, our mother or caretaker would instantly shove a bottle in our mouths. If it wasn't a bottle, it was a pacifier, which to our infant minds took the place of nourishment. I don't blame any of us for desiring that instant gratification when it comes to food, as it is ingrained in our psyche. We are very lucky to be living in a time of such great abundance that for most of us it is routinely possible to indulge in this way.

However, this concept means that you must be acutely sensitive to the end result, whether it be better health, or weight loss, or both. And it is this end result that must be foremost in your mind. We must have a much larger sense of responsibility to our eating habits than ever before in the history of mankind, simply because so many of our basic health needs can be taken for granted.

We have learned how to delay gratification in so many areas of our lives, but often do not delay when it comes to food. If we want a particular food, then we go get it. As a former overweight person, I can tell you I often have to resist giving in to my temptations and satisfying the immediate need. I desire being thin and healthy so much that I can give up whatever food I know I shouldn't have—at least most of the time. (After all, I'm only human like everybody else.)

You must let nothing stand in the way of attaining your goal. When that goal becomes the most important thing in your life, delaying instant gratification becomes a very easy thing to do. The end result becomes so much more important to you than that piece of cake, that bowl of white pasta, that white-flour bagel.

After all, know that the food you crave is not going anywhere. Those potato chips, that cupcake, Aunt Mary's cannolis, will all still be around six months from now, a year from now. Those foods will not disappear from the planet if you don't have them NOW.

*Learn to delay the gratification you get from food.* This will be a sure-fire way to deal with food cravings in the short term and maintain your new lower weight in the long term.

# CHAPTER 15

# The Mind-Body Medicines and Meal Plans—Week 3

The third week is when most people begin to give up on their diet. For some this may be the hardest week of dieting. However, I'm sure you are not about to do that, because you have the necessary tools, not only in knowing which foods to eat and which to avoid, but in having these mind-body medicines. Keep up the good work and don't stop now.

## Day 15

### Menu Suggestions

| | |
|---|---|
| Breakfast: | Artichoke Roll-Up |
| Lunch: | Vegas Strips |
| Dinner: | Salad of fresh arugula, radicchio, and endive with Italian Dressing |
| | Stuffed Chicken Breasts |
| Dessert: | Heidi's Sorbet |

### DAILY DOSE:
### *Thinness must be created.*

This is an important concept because you may want to be thin and just not know how. You think that just because you follow a diet you will become thin.

There is only one basic rule to being a thinner you, and that is creating it. This is the one concept I think most dieters miss. Being thin, at least for most of us, is not something that is going to come easily to us.

We have created our weight problem, either by eating the wrong foods, by not exercising, or by having some excuse or another why dieting is not as important as indulging. By the same token, we can create thinness. Even those born with the thin gene must learn how to eat correctly. This diet is appropriate for you, too. In the Western world, most of us learn how not to eat. It's time we learned the appropriate foods to eat, no matter if we are thin or not. By creating the possibility that we can be thin, we can then allow ourselves to remain that way for an extended period of time.

Many people come into my office feeling defeated from having tried so many diets in the past. They truly believe they will never be able to complete my diet, or if they can complete it successfully, manage to stay thin for any length of time. Being thin is not a concept that is familiar to them.

We have to learn a whole new way of being. We have to learn how to think like a thin person. We have to learn new ways of dining out, new ways of relating to parties, and new ways of being social, and that's just the tip of the iceberg. We have to create a new way of living our lives. This is tough, but not impossible. Half the battle is knowing we must do those things in order to be successful. That makes it that much easier.

I encourage you to try to see yourself as a thin person. Do this every day—in the car, when you are exercising, whenever you can. *Visualize yourself as a thin person, start thinking like one, and thereby create the possibility that being thin can happen to you.*

# Day 16

## Menu Suggestions

| | |
|---|---|
| Breakfast: | Florentine Omelet |
| Lunch: | Pretty in Pink |
| Dinner: | Rosemary-Scented Zucchini Soup |
| | V's Arrosto Di Vitello |
| Dessert: | 2 Peanut Butter Cookies |

### DAILY DOSE:
### *You must have more than a momentary commitment to being thinner.*

Many of my patients stay on their diets, make the necessary commitment for extended periods of time, and then at some point simply get tired and give up. They revert to their old habits. This can never happen if you want to stay thin for the rest of your life. The commitment must be lifelong.

I know this may be a scary concept, but commitment is of the utmost importance. There are definite reasons why people get so frightened about having to make the necessary commitments to succeed on a diet. After all, it is not just in dieting that this happens; it happens to us in many other aspects of our lives. Fear of commitment is something many men get accused of. But when it comes to dieting, believe me, women are just as bad as men.

Many of us just can't seem to make the necessary commitment, and I think in dieting it comes down to one simple thing: the fear of letting go of the comfortable. Many overweight people are comfortable in their bodies, either consciously or subconsciously. They become used to dealing with the world with whatever appearance they have. This is how we define our-selves, and if a change in that appearance comes, many of us simply don't know how to act. We need a new definition and being thin just doesn't fit right. It makes us extremely uncomfortable. It's like starting a new job. We don't know what to expect. However, like starting a new job, the unfamiliar quickly becomes familiar, and we can excel. The same should happen with dieting and becoming a thinner you. Don't let the unfamiliar stop you from being the person you want to be.

When you are thinking of cheating, or if you just need some encour-agement to remain on the diet, think of this daily dose and strive to have a commitment that lasts more than the moment. Make a commitment you will be proud of, one that will lead you to a lifetime of good health. Make the commitment, stick to it, and know that it is all right to be afraid of the unfa-miliar. *Acknowledge that negative feeling. Know that it is there and that it is nat-ural, and don't allow it to undermine your success.*

# Day 17

## Menu Suggestions

Breakfast:  Corned Beef Hash
Lunch:      Babe's Cod Salad
Dinner:     Stuffed Mushrooms
            Lamb Chops with Mint Butter
            Minted Quinoa

### DAILY DOSE:
### *Your desire to be thin can only be achieved through positive behaviors.*

The only way you can ever be thinner or healthier is by making proper decisions about which behaviors you want to take part in. The desire to be thin or healthy is a thought. The only way to make this thought a reality is through positive behaviors that will lead to that outcome. Thoughts do not become reality just because we think them. If they did we'd have real trou-ble on our hands. Yet when we think negative thoughts, especially around food, they so easily become reality.

Think about anything you have ever wanted in your life. If you are like most of us, you got those things through hard work. Most of us have had dreams, aspirations, and fantasies. How many of us have made those things come true?

Sneaking that piece of candy, having more vegetables than you should, indulging in too many nuts—these are not positive behaviors in terms of this diet because they don't lead to the outcome you wish to achieve. It's okay to think those thoughts but they cannot become actions or behaviors because they are not positive ways of being and will not lead to the outcome you desire.

This simple statement can make dieting really easy, because if the behavior you are contemplating does not lead you to attain the desire to be thin or healthy, the behavior is not something that you will do.

Ask yourself this question: Will the action I'm contemplating move me toward my goal or away from it? If the answer is away, the behavior should not be pursued. It's that simple.

Don't make becoming thinner or healthier another one of those thoughts or ideas that do not become reality. Many people, especially those of us who have suffered from chronic obesity, think being thin is an unattainable goal. It is not; we just have to adjust the way we think about getting there. This book and the program outlined here are only the tools to help you lose weight and get healthier. You are the one who is going to keep yourself thin by doing the necessary behaviors and making the necessary changes to get yourself there.

The next time you are standing in front of the refrigerator thinking about doing the wrong thing, remember this simple statement, and never do anything that will keep you from the important goal of attaining thinness and health.

# Day 18

## Menu Suggestions

| | |
|---|---|
| Breakfast: | Italian Roll-Up |
| Lunch: | Classic Chicken Melt |
| Dinner: | Arugula with Lemon and Caper Dressing |
| | Herbed Pork Scallops |
| Dessert: | 1 Fudge Brownie |

### DAILY DOSE:
### *There can be NO limitations in our consciousness to get thinner and healthier.*

We cannot go through a day focusing on the things we cannot achieve. If we do, we are setting the day up for failure before we have even gotten out of bed.

This is not to say that if I wanted to swim the English Channel tomorrow I could. But I know that if I wanted to train to do such a thing, I could at least accomplish that much.

We can have no limitations to what we can conceive, especially in terms of dieting. Far too often, we limit ourselves to thinking that there is no way we can ever go to this birthday party and stay on our diet, go out to dinner with friends and stay on our diet; get through the holidays and stay on our diet . . . and so on. I want you to list some of the things you think you cannot do while dieting:

1. _____

2. _____

3. _____

4. _____

I could never have been successful with myself or my patients if I thought there were any limitations.

I think one of the main reasons why patients enjoy seeing me as their physician is that I always look for different ways for them to stay on their diet, take their supplements, do whatever is necessary to get healthier. I never quit, because I truly believe there is no limitation to what we can achieve if we give it our best shot. If you fall down, you just get up again and keep trying. This attitude becomes contagious, and that is something my patients really enjoy and appreciate. I don't set any limits on myself, and I don't set any on my patients or on you.

Many people begin diets and never really expect in their heart of hearts that they are going to be successful. Or if they are successful, they don't really expect to be able to do it for the rest of their lives. They have all kinds of excuses: "My whole family is fat," "All my friends are overweight," "My spouse is not supportive enough," "I'm just big-boned." Whatever the excuse, the limitation is something you constructed. You have decided that the weight loss is not fast enough, you can't do this for another month. How come everyone else loses weight faster than me? It's you who have set up these obstacles and limitations. And you can just as easily remove them, because there can be no limitations in our consciousness if we are ever going to achieve our goal of losing weight and getting healthy.

Whenever you use this mind-body medicine, know that the limitation is something that you have constructed, then tear it right down, and know that you can get thin and healthy.

# Day 19

## Menu Suggestions

Breakfast:  New Wave Omelet
Lunch:      Minted Lamb Salad
Dinner:     Cauliflower and Cheddar Soup
            Herb Strip Steaks

DAILY DOSE:
*Ego is our only limitation in our quest for better health.*

You probably think that it is your ego that makes you want to be on a diet in the first place, that ego is the driving force that makes you want to look good. That may be true, but ego may also play a detrimental role in the dieting process.

Ego is what gets in the way of being able to say no to that cake, no to the dinner party invitation, no to your mother, no to the host of the dinner party you did go to. Most of us have to look good, no matter what, and I don't mean in a physical sense. We have to look good in the eyes of others, no matter the adverse outcome it may have in our lives. This is what I mean by ego.

Looking good in the eyes of others often takes precedence over our desire to lose weight and be healthy. This is a behavior pattern we must change. We must realize that "looking good" is not as important as being committed to our new diet and lifestyle program. The other people in our lives will have to understand the changes we are making and either they will help us or they will not. Those who are not helpful may be friends or family; if they are, then you're probably not going to be able to see them in social situations anymore. I know it sounds harsh, but if you are ever going to be truly successful, that is what needs to happen, at least for now. This is not to say that these people have to be cut out of your life. Far from it. This simply means that these people may have to play a different role in your life from the one you may be used to, at least while you are dieting.

For example, I am unable to have meals with my parents any longer, unless we go to a restaurant, because they have no limitations on the amount of food that can be consumed at any one sitting. My mother cooks more food than should ever be eaten at a meal and then she expects me to finish it all. And when I don't, she gets angry with me. To avoid that situation, I always ask that we see each other not at mealtimes, or at a restaurant where there are external portion controls. (I'm not sure she even realizes this, but I guess I let the cat out of the bag now!)

I'll give you another example of something I did when I used to try to lose weight on a regular basis. I scheduled events with my friends that involved doing things other than eating. We would go to the movies or go bowling—anything that did not involve food. I mention this only because mealtime is such a social event that people often feel that they can't enjoy the meal without imbibing or going along with the crowd. If your ego can't tolerate fitting in while being different, then I suggest you find other social activities to do with your friends and family that do not involve food. If you give it some thought, I'm sure you can come up with plenty of other common everyday things that can be shared that don't involve the worship of Bacchus: walking in the park, going to the museum, whatever.

*Use ego to your advantage, rather than having your ego destroy you and sabotage your good work.*

# Day 20

## Menu Suggestions

Breakfast: Poached Eggs on Greens
Lunch:     Bangkok Burger
Dinner:    Cheese Balls
           Veal Piccate
           Fancied-Up Brown Rice

### DAILY DOSE:
### *We must constantly battle to overcome our nature to eat the wrong foods.*

We do not like to change our patterns, even if those patterns are self-destructive and do nothing but cause us problems. We must overcome the wrong patterns and habits we learned about food when we were younger, and try to establish a brand new set of eating behaviors.

One of the toughest things I have to do with patients is convince them they may have to shop at a different place to buy lunch or groceries. This brings dread and fear into the lives of most people. I know it sounds funny, but it is not. Such changes cause very real problems for people, primarily because we are such creatures of habit. We hate to create new patterns. Yet that is what we must do if we are ever going to be successful dieters and keep the weight off for an extended period of time, preferably a lifetime.

This is the hardest one of the mind-body medicines to follow perfectly. Habits are extremely difficult things to break. If you've ever tried to quit smoking, you know what I mean. Well, that is easy compared to trying to change a food behavior. I have been thin for many years now, but my food thoughts are the same as they were when I was an overweight teenager. My habits are different, but only because I have to try extremely hard to change them. I have learned over the course of many years what I can get away with and what I can't, and constantly battle my inner self when it tells me to eat the wrong things. If it weren't so important to me to be thin, I would immediately revert to many of my former poor eating habits without batting an eyelash. That is how ingrained our food behaviors are.

Each of us will have a different demon to fight on a daily basis. But you have to know that you can overcome your nature, and that is easier to do when you know that it's a battle that must be waged on an ongoing basis. It is not something that is going to go away. You may think "OK, I lost the weight, when is my craving for the wrong foods going to go away?"

These feelings may never go away, so you're going to have to know that you can deal with them successfully. You have to win. The only way to win is to let go of your old patterns of living your life. Establish healthier new patterns by knowing that unhealthy behaviors may come from an unhealthy pattern, not out of a true need. That makes this a lot easier to understand and a lot easier to put into practice.

This mind-body medicine is the one that requires the most practice, so I encourage you to put it on an index card and carry it around with you, even if you have put none of the others on a card.

# Day 21

## Menu Suggestions

Breakfast: Benedict for the New Millennium
Lunch:     Taj Mahal
Dinner:    Spinach Salad with Oriental Dressing
           Stuffed Pork Loin
Dessert:   1 Mini Sour Cream Cheesecake

### DAILY DOSE:
### *What do I need to learn from being overweight?*

Ask yourself, What does food mean to me? What do I use food for other than nourishment so my body can perform the functions it needs to perform in a given day?

Take a few moments to write down in the space below all the things food means to you.

1. _____
2. _____
3. _____
4. _____

I'll give you an example. For me, food makes me happy, cheers me up when I am sad, gives me comfort when I've had a bad day, gives me something to do when I am bored. I encourage you to write down some psychological reasons that may even be painful. If we can face what there is to learn, maybe we have a chance to get rid of our eating problem forever.

We are given opportunities for growth in any situation in which we find ourselves, including being overweight or unhealthy. We need to reach inside and try to figure out what we need to learn, what we lack in our lives. These questions may lead you to the biggest breakthroughs you may ever have as a dieter—the answer to a lifetime of food abuse.

Have you ever said, "I was doing so well until . . . " Today's daily dose can help you figure out why that opportunity turned up. I want you to take a moment and write some things down about diets that you have been on in the past: I was doing so well until . . .

1. _____

2. _____

3. _____

4. _____

What do these situations have in common? I would bet there is an underlying theme and it is probably the one area in your life that dieting made most difficult. For me, it was being with my parents, and I have learned to handle that situation by never being with them at mealtimes. Is that the correct thing? Is that what I was supposed to learn? I don't know, but it works. I am not telling you that you need to go through an entire soul-searching experiment when it comes to weight loss. I only want to give you the tools you need to help create the new you, the one you are going to live with for many more years to come. That takes work. It is not easy, but I want you to do it.

Next time you find yourself inexplicably driven to the bakery, try to fig-ure out what is going on in your life and why you are really there. I will bet that it is not really because you want that fruit tart.

# CHAPTER 16

# The Mind-Body Medicines and Meal Plans—Week 4

Can you believe you've made it this far? I knew you could. Now there's just one more week to go and then you can proudly declare you've been dieting for one month.

Because you have done so well, this week is going to be nine days long, so that you will have an entire thirty days of menus and mind-body medicine in the form of daily doses in order to begin your new lifestyle program on the right foot.

This is the home stretch, so don't give up now. Things should be getting much easier. Your new program should be becoming much more routine—what may have seemed so foreign to you just three short weeks ago is now a part of your life. So let's go for it!

## Day 22

### *Menu Suggestions*

> Breakfast: Asian Omelet
> Lunch: Lemon Tarragon Chicken Salad
> Dinner: Squash Medley
> Classic Salmon
> Dessert: 2 Nut Gems

### DAILY DOSE:
### *Inject certainty into the dieting situation.*

Now that you have entered the home stretch, you should be absolutely certain that success is yours. I realize that you may be starting to get bored with the whole concept of dieting, and want to revert to your old, negative ways. Just remember that those emotions never worked for you at any time in the past, so why would they start working now? Don't be afraid of your success. Be certain that you will succeed. After all, frustration with your weight is something you've lived with all your life. Use that emotional level of dieting to your advantage. Be certain that this new way of eating is the best thing that has ever happened to you.

Certainty elevates your commitment to the next level. We have all been certain of some things in our lives, and if you think back to those times, you'll see they are when you have always succeeded. Maybe it was in a sports program as a kid, exams in school, bake contests at the local PTA. Whatever it is, you know that you excel at something, and you approach that something with absolute certainty. *There is no one better than me at . . .* And you succeed at that task, no matter what, because you know you are going to get through it—there is just no doubt in your mind.

I want you to write down something you feel you do better than anyone else. It can be anything, even something you consider really stupid. Don't be embarrassed. Remember, you're the only one who's going to be looking at this:

I am really good at . . .

1. _____
2. _____
3. _____
4. _____

Imagine being able to go through your entire life feeling the way you do when you do those things. It would be great, wouldn't it? All you have to do is try to refocus some of that really positive strength you get from being certain about those things you do really well into dieting.

This may be difficult if you have been a notoriously bad dieter. You lost the weight and then it went back on. How can you be certain that this time it is going to be a success when all the other times it hasn't?

You have never had my daily doses of mind-body medicine to combat all the psychological pitfalls that accompany dieting. And that's why you should not be so certain of failure. Instead, each day, you must be absolutely certain that you are not going to cheat. Think about how empowering that can be if you know there is no way you are going to do any of the wrong dieting things.

Even if you don't have the confidence to be certain you're going to be a successful dieter this time, just take it in stages and be certain you're not going to cheat today.

Doubt disappears, and serenity is there because you know only good is going to come out of each new day. I think many dieters live in constant fear of each new day, because that may be the day they are going to start doing all the wrong things. They think negatively—"Maybe this is going to be the day I screw up." This approach takes the power away from the dieter. Knowing for certain that this day is going to be a good day puts the power back in your hands. No one can take that away from you because you have control over what you eat and you are certain you are going to eat all the right things.

If there is any doubt—doubt that you could ever maintain this way of eating for the rest of your life or doubt that you could make it through another week—replace it with the certainty that you will be a success. Just know it! When faced with a poor food choice—something that you have given up for the past three weeks—and you can't see any way around eating it, *you must be confident enough in yourself to know for certain that you are not going to eat it.* The desire will then practically vanish.

When you are faced with improper food decisions and you think this is the end and you can see no way out, know for certain (beyond a shadow of a doubt, as if your life depended on it) *that there is a way out, that it is the right way, and you will succeed.*

# Day 23

## Menu Suggestions

Breakfast:  Greek Roll-Up
Lunch:  Diana
Dinner:  Eastern Tofu or Lemon Flowers
           Horseradish Chicken
           Nutty Grain

### DAILY DOSE:
### *Don't do all the right, healthy things for the wrong reasons.*

You may say "If I am dieting, what difference does it make why I do it if I still lose weight?" This may be all right for the weight loss section of the diet, but can never be good enough for the maintenance section of the diet. It may never be good enough even for the weight loss section of the diet, because if it were good enough, then why are you reading yet another diet book? Why haven't all the other diet books worked for you?

The reason is that the other diet books never showed you how to achieve a proper mind-body balance after the weight loss was achieved. Those other books never gave you this exceptional program to help you overcome your worst dieting obstacles. You must begin to make the correct food choices and make the correct mind choices for the right reasons.

So what is the right reason? To be honest, I don't think you can always tell what the truly right reasons are. I know what some of the wrong reasons are: losing weight for your spouse, losing weight for your mother, losing weight because you should, losing weight because you're getting older—the list goes on. There is no way you can even hope to achieve long-term success with those wrong reasons in place. I want you to write down a few reasons why you're trying to lose weight.

1. _____
2. _____
3. _____
4. _____

It is important that we work backwards from our goal. First we must establish a goal and then do everything necessary to reach that goal. Nothing should stand in our way. We can let nothing make us veer from our path. We can't be wishy-washy when it comes to having a goal. We either have one or we don't. I think most of us, at least when it comes to dieting, think that if we don't succeed today, there will be another day, the next diet, the next goal to set. How many of us also wake up twenty years later and realize that not only are we not in the same place we were then, but we are actually far worse because the 20 pounds we had to lose then have now ballooned to 50?

You must have the right reasons for losing weight—like doing it for yourself or doing it to get over a feeling of inadequacy you lived behind all your life because of your weight. The right reasons are probably going to be quite deep and complex. Something that may take some work, something you may not want to explore. But I know that exploration is worth the effort, and it will help make this diet the last diet you will ever need.

# Day 24

## Menu Suggestions

Breakfast:  Spinach Pie
Lunch:      Louisiana Burger
Dinner:     Lemon Asparagus
            Jamaican Pork Chops

### DAILY DOSE:
*The path of least resistance to do the wrong thing is often the most chaotic.*

How many times have you chosen to take the easy way out only to find that it caused more problems than it was worth? How many times have you chosen the cheaper solution to a problem only to have the job wind up costing you more in the end?

These are things we have all experienced at one time or another, but have you ever thought about them in terms of dieting? Think about this scenario: You're out to dinner and your companion suggests you share a dessert. You know you're on a diet, but your companion says, "Oh, it's just this once" or "How can a forkful make a difference?" So, to save face, or to get out of an awkward confrontation, you go along with your dinner mate, and then spend the next few hours/days/minutes regretting what you've done and trying to figure out ways of making this situation right.

Worse yet, this one forkful can sometimes be the trigger for a dieter to completely abandon a diet, surely leading to the road to chaos. And why? Simply because you chose the path of least resistance. Chaos may seem like a funny word to you, but if you think about it, it makes perfect sense. What you are doing when you make that incorrect food choice will absolutely make your life a lot more difficult, more chaotic, and possibly even more traumatic—depending on how much guilt you let yourself live with. Giving in may look easier at the outset, but as you can see, it definitely isn't easier once you do it. I often refer to this as the slippery slope. Once you start down that road, watch out. Nothing is safe. Fasten your seat belts, it's going to be a bumpy night in front of the refrigerator.

Never make the easy decision to give in to temptation. Never accept that dinner party invitation if you can't have certainty that you will be able to stay on your diet. Never go out for drinks with your friends if you know you are probably going to partake of the alcohol and you are not yet up to that phase of the diet.

*Don't make your life any more difficult than it has to be. Follow the rules and stay the course.*

# Day 25

## Menu Suggestions

Breakfast: Corned Beef Hash
Lunch: Chicken Licken
Dinner: Lettuce Salad with Italian Dressing
         Chicken and Sausage Bundles
Dessert: Lemon Cheesecake Square

### DAILY DOSE:
### *What am I supposed to learn from this bagel?*

We should approach most situations as if we need to learn something from them. Our reaction to any given situation can be more controlled if we take the time to figure out the thing we need to learn. That piece of chocolate, that bagel, becomes so much less important if we see it as a challenge to overcome. Why did one of the women at the office decide on the day you were starting your diet to bring in a box of donuts? Why did your husband decide that the day you were starting your diet was the day he wanted to take you out to a fancy restaurant for dinner?

Did you ever wonder why something happens to you seemingly out of the blue? Why did you run into that particular person? Why did you get that letter on that day? I look at these situational events in our lives and think that there must be a reason why these things happen to us.

I want you to try an exercise I learned a while ago. Get a pen and paper. Now think back to three times in your life: growing up as a child, your first relationship, and something that happened to you recently or is happening to you now. Think of the events that bothered you the most during those times in your life. Write them down:

1. _____
2. _____
3. _____

What things had a profound impact on how you felt each time? The things you remember probably affected you deeply. Write them down on a separate piece of paper and try to figure out what they have in common. I can guarantee there will be a commonality.

It is this common thread we are trying to overcome when we are placed in any difficult situation. How does this relate to dieting? Whenever we are given the opportunity to eat the wrong things, we are put in that situation for a reason.

We can either try to figure out why, or we can just remove ourselves from the situation without ever trying to figure out the reason. Either way, the bottom line remains the same: get yourself out of what is a bad deal. If you try to figure out the root cause, this will significantly help your ability to stay on this and any other diet you may try in the future.

That's a great incentive to try to do the work it takes to figure it all out. The need to "diet" will disappear, and the thinner and healthier you will be around for the rest of your life, without your even having to think about it.

# Day 26

## Menu Suggestions

Breakfast: Southwest Omelet
Lunch: Janis
Dinner: Spinach with Pine Nuts
Fourth of July Chicken
Dessert: Snickersnoo

## DAILY DOSE:
### *You are responsible to others, not for others—*
### *don't use them as an excuse.*

As dieters, we often look to others to give us an excuse for what we do wrong. "My wife made me do it." "It's my husband's fault I'm fat." "I needed to keep that food in the house for my kids." How many of these excuses and countless others have you used over and over again?

Yes, we have to be responsible to the other people in our lives. I am not advocating that you ignore your family and friends because you are on a diet. What I am saying is that you cannot let their needs supersede yours, nor should you let their needs be an excuse for you to do the wrong things. Let's remove that excuse from the picture right now.

We do not have to be responsible for other people's actions, for what they eat. This feeling of responsibility is another level of guilt, another level of stuff we add to our daily lives that just doesn't need to be there. We take the way these things make us feel, turn it against ourselves, then use it as today's reason to do the wrong thing, or as the reason why we can never be on this or any diet for any length of time.

Sometimes we feel that because others around us are not on the same diet we are getting no support, or there will be too many temptations in the house. All it means is that the rest of our family is on a different diet from the one we are on. They are eating differently. It doesn't make you right and them wrong. It has no meaning other than the fact that they are eating different foods from the foods you are. Do not ascribe any more meaning to it than that.

As for the "temptations" that are in the house, they are foods—they are only temptations if you make them temptations. They are just bagels, or just chocolate, or whatever you find particularly troublesome. Don't make them what they are not.

Be responsible for your own actions, not for the actions of others. They are not making you do anything. And you are certainly not responsible for their behaviors. Don't add this level of guilt to so many others you may be experiencing. Today's simple thought will help you get through some difficult times in your dieting career.

# Day 27

## Menu Suggestions

Breakfast: Traditional Roll-Up
Lunch: Veneto
Dinner: Baked Okra
Baked Eggplant
Dessert: Creamy Watermelon Frozen Dessert

## DAILY DOSE:
### *No pain, no gain.*

You were probably wondering when this one was going to show up. I think it's a perfect thought for the end of a very rewarding month of dieting, the beginning of the road to forever. You have to accept this simple fact: you will never get anything that is worthwhile without working for it. There may be some suffering involved, but it will all be worth it in the long run.

Although this is one concept I'm sure many of you are familiar with, how many of us actually have the guts to do what it takes to be a successful dieter? How many of us are able to go through our daily lives making the necessary sacrifices?

Believe me, I know how difficult it is to stay the course. I have been dieting for over twenty years, and it does get easier but it never gets easy. The pain associated with dieting is psychological, almost never physiological. Don't let the mental anguish tear you down. Besides, with all these daily doses of mind-body medicine, you now have most of the tools you need so that you never have to experience the frustration of not being a successful dieter.

# Day 28

## *Menu Suggestions*

Breakfast: Ham and Eggs
Lunch:    Carly
Dinner:    Southwest Tofu or Sesame Spinach
           Cornish Game Hens
           Kasha Salad

## DAILY DOSE:
### *If the reward is any good, you've got to earn it.*

The amount of energy you put into something, especially dieting, is the amount of reward you will usually reap. This is the psychological component to "no pain, no gain." This mind-body medicine is the psychological work necessary to get us to the next level. Nothing good is ever easy to achieve or to maintain. Being on a diet is hard work, and so is staying the course long after the initial thrill has worn off, long after the initial rewards are no longer felt, long after you've gotten used to the new, improved, thinner you.

Many people get bored with the concept of dieting. They feel they can go back to their old ways of eating and their old ways of being once they have lost weight. Not true. Now that you have lost the weight, the fun is just beginning. You've worked really hard. There is no other way, if you want to attain anything worthwhile. Now comes your opportunity to continue that good work. Now you are going to reap the largest rewards, because now you are able to make changes and keep the changes you have made and make a significant difference in your overall health and well-being. The weight loss is nothing compared to the rest of the benefits you are going to see from an improved way of eating.

All too often, patients forget what they looked like when they first came into the office, or they forget how bad they were feeling because it's been such a long time since they felt that way. I like to take pictures of my patients when they first come in to remind them of what they looked like when they began the program.

By staying on this diet through the twenty-eighth day, you have made great changes in the way you eat, more than likely. You have earned the reward, so don't let all that good work slip away.

By this point, you have made huge strides against heart disease, diabetes, high blood pressure, and other major illnesses just by losing weight and getting rid of most of the sugar in your life. Don't blow it now because you feel you have come to the end. This is not the end, it is just the beginning.

# Day 29

## Menu Suggestions

| | |
|---|---|
| Breakfast: | Which Came First? |
| Lunch: | Velvety Chicken Soup |
| Dinner: | Brussels Sprouts Italiano |
| | Grilled Veal Chops |
| Dessert: | Crepes du Jour |

### DAILY DOSE:
### *You are in this dieting game, play it for all it's worth.*

Think of dieting as a game. As long as you've decided to play the game, don't you want to play it to win? I think most of us tend to take dieting far too seriously. Dieting becomes this mysterious thing that we think others can do well and we can't. Nothing is further from the truth.

We are all bad at dieting, and that's why there is a multibillion-dollar dieting industry in North America today. Most of us think that dieting is something that is done to us and that we don't have to play an active role. We think that if we read such and such a book, that will be the answer. That may help, but the answer to a lifetime of yo-yo dieting comes from you and only from you. It comes from the inside. That's where your thin person resides—in your mind. My diet provides you with the important mind-body tools you are going to need to carry this program further and to bring that inner thin person to the forefront. You've lost weight and I wholeheartedly congratulate you. However, now is not the time to stop and indulge yourself. Now is the time to make preparations so that this great success will continue.

You can make all the necessary changes to your life in order to win this game. You have all the components you need right now in order to keep the excess weight off forever. You just have to change the way you think about dieting. Be competitive—not with others, but with yourself. It's not a team effort, like baseball or football. It's like bowling or golf or some other individual sport you prefer. You have to do this on your own. Play to win. Try to better your personal best. Give it your best shot, and mean it. Make your words and your thoughts mean something by being successful.

*Play this game as if your life depended on it, because, quite frankly, it may.*

# Day 30

## Menu Suggestions

Breakfast:  Shrimp Surprise Roll-Up
Lunch:       Taxco Topper
Dinner:      Dressed-Up Cauliflower
               Beefsteaks with Gorgonzola Sauce

### DAILY DOSE:
### *You will always be that overweight person.*

The end of the initiation diet is the perfect place to discuss this concept. It is something I've touched upon throughout this book, but I feel you deserve a full explanation of the concept. *Remember that the initiation phase of the diet may take longer than these thirty days. It all depends on how much weight you need to lose.*

This is not meant to sound harsh, defeatist, or even remotely negative. Instead, this is as empowering as any of the other mind-body doses that have come before it. It may actually hold more power than many of them combined.

You must know that losing weight and feeling better about yourself is not going to change your life. You are not going to become someone other than who you are simply by being successful on this program. Yes, you will be thinner, and this is a great accomplishment. However, even though the outside of you might change, inside you are going to be the same person.

I am hoping that, like many of my patients, you will be able to use these daily doses to make some permanent changes in your life. That is what they are designed to do. They have certainly made permanent changes in my life, and not only when it comes to being thinner. They have helped in other areas too.

What I'm really talking about is the person you see when you look into a mirror. More than likely, that person will always be overweight. That doesn't mean you should give up and just physically be that overweight person. I am that overweight person and yet on the outside, I am thin. I don't want you to think that just because externally you are now thinner that you automatically become the thinner person internally. This will take time—how long I can't say. What I do know is that for me it's been twenty years and it still hasn't changed.

I want you to be able to accept this fact without using it as an excuse to revert to your old eating ways. Accepting the fact can have a profound impact on your future. This acceptance empowers you to do the right things, make the right food decisions, and do everything I've been talking about.

Don't expect your entire life to change once you've lost weight. Be prepared to have a struggle ahead of you that is difficult, but infinitely rewarding. My struggle with these issues has enabled me to dedicate my life to helping others get out of the web of obesity and to helping children avoid a lifetime of weight issues. It has been rewarding for me and I know it can be equally as rewarding for you. Good luck. I know you can do it.

## The Thin For Good Rules

Now that you know what my mind-body medicines are, the only other thing you need to do to be a successful dieter is to follow and acknowledge these ten simple rules:

Rule 1: Maintaining a weight loss is never easy.

Rule 2: Don't believe any diet book that says it is.

Rule 3: You can lose weight on most any diet. The key to being a successful dieter is keeping the weight off.

Rule 4: Each daily dose of mind-body medicine may be used once, more than once, or not at all.

Rule 5: Use the ones that work best for you.

Rule 6: Make an index card with each day's dose written in bold letters. If necessary, make multiple cards and keep them in such trouble spots as on the refrigerator, in the car, at the office, and in your pocket.

Rule 7: Refer to this index card constantly throughout the day, especially when you feel a hunger craving coming on, or find yourself in a difficult dieting situation.

Rule 8: Don't beat yourself up.

Rule 9: The daily doses are not optional.

Rule 10: Have fun!

# CHAPTER 17

# Eight Weeks to Thin For Good: The Forever Phase

If you adhere to the rules set forth in this chapter you will be able to keep off the weight you've lost. Forever. I know, every diet book says the same thing, but if you allow yourself to follow these simple guidelines, you can truly be thinner for the rest of your life.

Women and men alike should read this chapter. Follow the instructions that pertain to what you have been doing in your initiation phase. This is quite simple to do and must be done if you want to continue to be successful.

There is no set time frame for staying on the diet outlined for your initiation phase. Some may need a whole month, whereas others will need two months or even a year. It all depends on how much weight you need to lose and how quickly you can accomplish your goal.

But remember this: losing weight is not a race against time. Most people who use time as their excuse for going off a diet are merely looking for a convenient out. I can appreciate the frustration they have, because of all the hard work a diet entails. The weight should just fly off, but what if it doesn't? Should you give up? Of course not. Instead, try to look at things from the top of the mountain, not the bottom. I'll give you a great example that happened just the day before I sat down to write this chapter.

Della came to my office for her routine checkup. It was the second time she had been back since starting the diet program. She was extremely distraught because she had tried so hard and had managed to lose only 4 pounds in the past month. In the prior month, she had lost 6 pounds, and even that was too slow for her. Della had about 75 pounds to lose, so she was very anxious for the process to go faster. I explained to her that in the past two months she had lost 10 pounds, not an insignificant amount of weight. Since she was averaging 5 pounds per month, 5 pounds times twelve months would equal 60 pounds in one year. When she looked at it this way—at the big picture—she was relieved and a little excited, and she was ready, even eager, to continue on the diet. When you read the mind-body medicines, you will see the dangers of bringing expectations to any dieting program. But you will also learn the tools to change this negative feeling into something that can work for you and not against you.

## Slowly but Surely

From the start, you must realize that the long-term plan I'm about to outline will be a slow process. This is the best way to achieve success and it provides another bonus, because in using a slower process you will be able to accomplish more than just weight loss. By going slowly, you will be able to accomplish a lifetime of success, not just a temporary weight loss that will have you back on a different diet a year from now.

The trick is this: When you are dieting, you should be learning how to eat new and different foods, or be learning how to eat these foods in a different way that allows you to still enjoy the foods you like without gaining the weight that you don't like. The more time you have to learn these new habits, the easier it will be to maintain them for the rest of your life. New habits take a long time to master. Think how long it takes to learn a new sport, or a new language as an adult. In this case, you are essentially learning a new language—the language of a new nutritional lifestyle program.

All too often, people think that once they have achieved their goal weight, they should be able to go back to the way they have always eaten. Nothing could be further from the truth. Imagine trying to do the same thing over and over while anticipating different results. This is what most of us do every time we try to diet. This is where the frustration comes in. This is what makes you think you can never be a successful dieter. This is what makes you angry. The mind-body program in my diet eliminates such frustrations. It puts you in the mood of weight loss. Be patient and take full advantage of the mind-body program. It is easier to break old habits when you know why you are doing them in the first place. When you can see what the bad habit is all about, you can see a way of changing it into a productive habit.

## Making the Transition to the New You

First of all, congratulations! You've made it this far in the program, and now you are down to the weight you want to be. That's great, but now what? The guidelines that follow will help you to figure out the best way to eat for a lifetime.

Every one of us is different, so the guidelines I am going to offer are those that have worked for the majority of my patients. They should be easy for you to follow whether you eat at home or eat out. The rules will be the same for each and every dieter, female and male, even for the vegetarians (the only difference for the vegetarians will come when I mention the proteins. Just refer to your particular types of proteins and the rest of the forever program will be the same). Here are a few general guidelines:

- Think of this phase in terms of weeks. Each week will allow you to add different foods.
- The amounts of foods that you add will be determined by which initiation phase stage you started in.
- The types of foods will be determined by you according to the rules I will set forth. You can eat the foods you like while still maintaining your dietary goal of keeping the weight off. You may want more vegetables in your diet, whereas your wife may want some more complex grains. This is entirely possible, because you will be essentially designing your own transition program within the guidelines.

## How Does the Transition Work?

Normally, the transition period should take eight weeks. It may not be exactly the same for each dieter, though, and you should be prepared to make some adjustments. The most common adjustment people have to make is that they must repeat a week, possibly more. For some, the transition period may take as long as sixteen weeks, for others up to a year. Unless you have another medical problem, you should be able to do well with the eight-week transition period. Again, just as in the initiation phase, each person's diet is unique and therefore the time frame will be unique as well. Please remember the eight-week schedule is not etched in stone—it's just a guideline.

Should you start to gain weight again during any particular week, go immediately to the preceding week's program and repeat it. Some patients may never be able to get out of the previous week's range, and that will be their forever phase. Some may never be able to add all the foods back to the diet that they would want in the amounts that they would want. There are many possible reasons for this. In coming chapters, I will describe some of these scenarios to remove another layer of frustration and uncertainty.

I want you to know that it is possible to get through all eight weeks no matter what; it's just that those eight weeks may take as long as a year to complete.

Here's the program.

# Week 1

This is the simplest week because it has the fewest options to add.

## Proteins

| | |
|---|---|
| **Red Meats** | The amounts remain the same. |
| **Processed Meats** | The amounts remain the same. |
| **Fish** | The amounts remain the same. |
| **Poultry** | The amounts remain the same. |
| **Eggs** | The amounts remain the same. |
| **Cheeses** | |
|    *Category 1:* | These may increase by 1 ounce each day. |
|    *Category 2:* | These may increase by 1 ounce each day. |

## Complex Carbohydrates

| | |
|---|---|
| **Vegetables** | |
|    *Category 1:* | These may increase by 1 cup each day. |
|    *Category 2:* | These may increase by ¼ cup each day. |
|    *Category 3:* | These remain the same. |
| **Grains** | These remain the same. |
| **Nuts and Seeds** | These remain the same. |
| **Legumes** | These remain the same. |

## Desserts

These remain the same.

## Condiments

These remain the same.

## Beverages

| | |
|---|---|
| **Alcohol** | These remain the same. |
| **Milk** | These remain the same. |

## Fruit

These remain the same.

# Week 2

## Proteins

| | |
|---|---|
| **Red Meats** | These remain the same. |
| **Processed Meats** | These remain the same. |
| **Fish** | These remain the same. |
| **Poultry** | These remain the same. |

| Eggs | For those on an egg restriction, eggs can now be unlimited. |
| Cheeses | These remain at the new levels described in week 1. |

## Complex Carbohydrates

**Vegetables**

| *Category 1:* | These can now be eaten in unlimited quantities. |
| *Category 2:* | You may add an additional ¼-cup serving each day *or* |
| *Category 3:* | You may add an additional ¼-cup serving three days each week. |

| **Grains** | You may add an additional ¼-cup cooked serving on the other three days of the week. |
| **Nuts and Seeds** | These remain the same. |
| **Legumes** | These remain the same. |

## Desserts

These remain the same.

## Condiments

These remain the same.

## Beverages

| Alcohol | An additional ounce of alcohol may be added to your allotment, from category 2, once each week. If alcohol is permitted here for the first time, then it can be had only once each week, 1 ounce from category 1. |
| Milk | These remain the same. |

## Fruit

These remain the same.

# Week 3

## Proteins

| **Red Meats** | These remain the same. |
| **Processed Meats** | These remain the same. |
| **Fish** | These remain the same. |
| **Poultry** | These remain the same. |
| **Eggs** | These remain the same. |

Cheeses
> *Category 1:*     These can be increased by 1 ounce each day over previous weeks; *or*
>
> *Category 2:*     These may be increased by 1 ounce each day.

## Complex Carbohydrates

**Vegetables**
> *Category 1:*     These remain the same.
>
> *Category 2:*     These may be increased by ¼-cup serving each day; *or*
>
> *Category 3:*     These may be increased to every day in the same quantity as the previous week.

**Grains**     These may be increased to every day *or* the allotted amount of whole grain bread may be increased to every day.

**Nuts and Seeds**     These remain the same.

**Legumes**     These remain the same.

## Desserts

These remain the same.

## Condiments

These remain the same.

## Beverages

**Alcohol**     For those just allowed alcohol from category 1: at this point, you may increase the amount by 2 ounces.

For those allowed alcohol from both category 1 and 2: you may add an additional day, but with the same amount, in ounces, as the previous week.

**Milk**     4 ounces nonsweetened, plain yogurt can be added twice per week; all else remains the same.

## Fruit

> *Category 1:*     This may be increased to an additional ½-cup serving two days each week, if previously allowed, and if not previously allowed, then ½-cup serving twice each week.
>
> *Category 2:*     These remain the same.
>
> *Category 3:*     These remain the same.
>
> *Category 4:*     These remain the same.

# Week 4

## Proteins

| | |
|---|---|
| Red Meats | These should be reduced by 1 ounce in each category; *or* |
| Processed Meats | These should be reduced by 1 ounce in each category; *or* |
| Fish | These should be reduced by 1 ounce in each category; *or* |
| Poultry | These should be reduced by 1 ounce in each category. |
| Eggs | These remain the same. |
| Cheeses | These remain the same. |

## Complex Carbohydrates

**Vegetables**

| | |
|---|---|
| *Category 1:* | These remain the same. |
| *Category 2:* | These may be increased by an additional ¼-cup serving each day. |
| *Category 3:* | These may be increased to every day, in the same serving size. |
| Grains | These remain the same. |
| Nuts and Seeds | These remain the same. |
| Legumes | For those who have been eating legumes, they may be increased by two days each week, in the same serving size. For the rest, they may be increased by ¼ cup three days each week. |

## Desserts

These remain the same.

## Condiments

These remain the same.

## Beverages

| | |
|---|---|
| Alcohol | These remain the same. |
| Milk | This remains the same. |

## Fruit

These remain the same.

# Week 5

## Proteins

| | |
|---|---|
| **Red Meats** | These remain the same. |
| **Processed Meats** | These remain the same. |
| **Fish** | These remain the same. |
| **Poultry** | These remain the same. |
| **Eggs** | These remain the same. |
| **Cheeses** | |
| *Category 1:* | These may be increased by 1 ounce each day; *or* |
| *Category 2:* | These may be increased by 1 ounce each day. |

## Complex Carbohydrates

| | |
|---|---|
| **Vegetables** | |
| *Category 1:* | These remain the same. |
| *Category 2:* | These may increase by ¼-cup serving each day. |
| *Category 3:* | These may increase to every day at the same serving size as the previous week. |
| **Grains** | These may increase by ¼-cup serving each day and may be had every day, *or* you may have 2 slices of whole grain bread each day. |
| **Nuts and Seeds** | |
| *Category 1:* | These remain the same. |
| *Category 2:* | These are now permitted up to a ½-ounce serving three times each week. |
| **Legumes** | These remain the same. |

## Desserts

These remain the same.

## Condiments

These remain the same.

## Beverages

| | |
|---|---|
| **Alcohol** | Is now permitted up to 4 ounces each day for those who have been more restricted, and now half may come from either category 1 or category 2. For those who have been allowed alcohol from the beginning, you may now have it an additional day each week, *or* you may have 2 ounces from category 3 up to twice each week. |
| **Milk** | This remains the same. |

## Fruit

| | |
|---|---|
| *Category 1:* | These remain the same. |
| *Category 2:* | These are allowed up to ½-cup serving once each week. |
| *Category 3:* | These remain the same. |
| *Category 4:* | These remain the same. |

# Week 6

## Proteins

| | |
|---|---|
| **Red Meats** | These should be decreased by 1 ounce in each category each day; *or* |
| **Processed Meats** | These should be decreased by 1 ounce in each category each day; *or* |
| **Fish** | These should be decreased by 1 ounce in each category each day; *or* |
| **Poultry** | These should be decreased by 1 ounce each day in each category. |
| **Eggs** | These remain the same. |
| **Cheeses** | |
| *Category 1:* | These may be increased by 1 ounce each day. |
| *Category 2:* | These may be increased by 1 ounce each day. |

## Complex Carbohydrates

| | |
|---|---|
| **Vegetables** | |
| *Category 1:* | These remain the same. |
| *Category 2:* | These remain the same. |
| *Category 3:* | These may increase by ¼-ounce serving each day. |
| **Grains** | These remain the same. |
| **Nuts and Seeds** | |
| *Category 1:* | These may increase by ½ ounce each day; *or* |
| *Category 2:* | These may increase to ½ ounce each day. |
| **Legumes** | These may now be increased to a daily serving in the same serving size as before. |

## Desserts

These remain the same.

## Condiments

These remain the same.

## Beverages

| | |
|---|---|
| Alcohol | These remain the same. |
| Milk | This remains the same. |

## Fruit

| | |
|---|---|
| *Category 1:* | These remain the same. |
| *Category 2:* | These may be increased to a ½-cup serving three times each week. |
| *Category 3:* | These remain the same. |
| *Category 4:* | These remain the same. |

# Week 7

## Proteins

| | |
|---|---|
| **Red Meats** | These remain the same. |
| **Processed Meats** | These remain the same. |
| **Fish** | These remain the same. |
| **Poultry** | These remain the same. |
| **Eggs** | These remain the same. |
| **Cheeses** | These remain the same. |

## Complex Carbohydrates

**Vegetables**

| | |
|---|---|
| *Category 1:* | These remain the same. |
| *Category 2:* | These are now permitted in unlimited quantities. |
| *Category 3:* | These remain the same. |
| **Grains** | The grains may increase in serving size by ¼ cup each day. The amount of bread remains the same. |

**Nuts and Seeds**

| | |
|---|---|
| *Category 1:* | These remain the same. |
| *Category 2:* | These may increase to 1 ounce each day. |
| **Legumes** | These may be increased by a ¼-cup serving each day. |

## Desserts

These remain the same.

## Condiments

These remain the same.

## Beverages

| | |
|---|---|
| Alcohol | You may now include category 3, wine or beer, twice each week, up to 4 ounces, regardless of where you started the dieting process. Category 1 and category 2 remain the same. |
| Milk | Yogurt can now be increased to 4 ounces 4 times per week. All else remains the same. |

## Fruit

| | |
|---|---|
| *Category 1:* | This may increase by a ½-cup serving every day; *or* |
| *Category 2:* | This may increase to a ½-cup serving every day. |
| *Category 3:* | These remain the same. |
| *Category 4:* | These remain the same. |

# Week 8

## Proteins

| | |
|---|---|
| **Red Meats** | These remain the same. |
| **Processed Meats** | These remain the same. |
| **Fish** | These remain the same. |
| **Poultry** | These remain the same. |
| **Eggs** | These remain the same. |
| **Cheeses** | These remain the same. |

## Complex Carbohydrates

**Vegetables**

| | |
|---|---|
| *Category 1:* | These remain the same. |
| *Category 2:* | These remain the same. |
| *Category 3:* | These may increase by a ¼-cup serving each day. |
| **Grains** | These remain the same. |

**Nuts and Seeds**

| | |
|---|---|
| *Category 1:* | The maximum allowed is 2 ounces each day; *or* |
| *Category 2:* | The maximum allowed is 2 ounces each day. |
| **Legumes** | These remain the same. |

## Desserts

These remain the same.

## Condiments

These remain the same.

## Beverages

| | |
|---|---|
| Alcohol | The 4 ounces of category 3 may now be increased to four times each week. All others remain the same. |
| Milk | This remains the same. |

## Fruit

| | |
|---|---|
| *Category 1:* | The maximum allowable is 1 cup each day; *or* |
| *Category 2:* | The maximum allowable is ¾ cup each day; *or* |
| *Category 3:* | The maximum allowable is ½ cup each day. |
| *Category 4:* | I think these fruits should be avoided at all times. However, if you would like to have the rare indulgence, then just make sure you have had no other fruit for that day. And make this a *rare* indulgence. |

Wasn't that easy and satisfying, and didn't you get great results? I offered all the different food choices, but I certainly don't expect you to indulge in every food choice I offered every day. Use the better judgment you've learned in the past few months as we've been dieting together. Make healthy choices from the many listings I've given you. Keep up the smaller portions of food if you can.

## Where to Go from Here

By the time you've been through all the phases of this diet, you should have found a comfortable level of eating without gaining any weight. I leave it up to you to determine where you need to be in terms of how much food you can eat. I can't predict how much you should be eating. Just use the guidelines above, and when you get to the last week you can manage without gaining weight, then you have reached your proper level, and this becomes your new and improved way of eating—your forever diet.

By the time you get to this point, you will be eating a meal that generally consists of 55 percent protein, 40 percent complex carbohydrates, and 5 percent simple carbohydrates, usually in the form of fruit. Your plate should always be balanced. Don't eat all your carbohydrates in the morning for breakfast. Balance each meal so that your body's metabolism runs at its most efficient level, and so that you feel your best.

Each meal should look something like this:

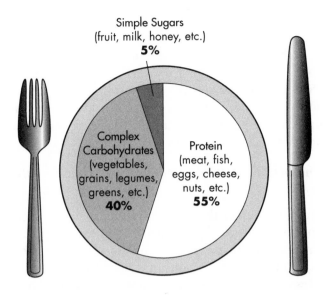

Simple Sugars
(fruit, milk, honey, etc.)
**5%**

Complex
Carbohydrates
(vegetables,
grains, legumes,
greens, etc.)
**40%**

Protein
(meat, fish,
eggs, cheese,
nuts, etc.)
**55%**

# Dr. Fred's Helpful Hints

Since no diet or dieter is perfect, you may encounter some problems along the way. I'd like to discuss the most common trouble spots I have seen in my years of practice so that you will know what to do should any of these arise for you. I do not want any of these possible problems to be your excuse for giving up. There are ways around most difficulties, so stick with it.

### My weight loss is slow. What's the problem?

First of all, think back to what I said about "slow" weight loss. Look at other factors, such as your health and how you are feeling. If they have improved, the diet has been successful.

Now let's think about some reasons your weight loss may be slow. I have found the most common reason to be that you're eating too much, especially in the really restricted categories of food. One ounce is not a lot. One-half cup is not that much food.

On the flip side, the second thing to look at is to see if you are eating enough. Sometimes people will go on extremely low-calorie diets when they try to lose weight. You may not be giving your body enough fuel to do its job, and this can often encourage your body to store calories because it thinks it is starving.

Underlying yeast infections can also be the cause of slow or no weight loss. If it is, I would place you on the yeast restricted version of the diet (see chapter 20). Certain prescription drugs, food allergies, an underactive thyroid, or a hormonal imbalance can all lead to a slower weight loss than you might expect. (Remember what I said about expectations.)

The fourth thing to look at is the water rule. Remember that you must make sure you are drinking enough water.

The fifth thing is to make sure you are doing some form of exercise.

And finally, some people are extremely sensitive to artificial sweeteners. Try to eliminate these products or, at the very least, limit them to the bare necessity and see if that does the trick.

### I've got some other medical conditions. Is this a problem on this diet?

I think you should be under the care of a physician before embarking on any weight-loss program, especially if you are taking any medications. There is no reason why you can't be on this diet, unless you have extremely advanced kidney disease, but your medications may need to be adjusted and probably lowered as a result of the beneficial response you will most likely have to this diet. This is especially true for people with diabetes.

### Are there any medications that may interfere with my ability to lose weight?

Yes. There is a long list, so I will list only the most common. These include the beta blockers, antidepressants, and hormone replacement therapy (including steroids, such as prednisone). If you are on any of these medications, you can still do the diet, but weight loss may just be more difficult. Whatever you do, do not go off any medications that you may be taking without the advice of your physician.

### Will I have problems if I drink coffee or black tea?

Yes. Caffeine will cause an overproduction of insulin in your body. As we are trying to regulate your insulin levels, I recommend you avoid these as much as you can.

### How about aspartame?

Aspartame may interrupt the way your brain works. That is why I recommend you avoid any products that contain this substance. However, I know that you won't, so try to keep your usage down to a minimum.

### Can my child go on this diet with me?

Children and adults have different metabolisms and therefore need to be on different diets. Please read my first book, *Feed Your Kids Well*, which is a health and nutrition book geared specifically for parents. The basics are quite similar, so there will not be that many conflicts at mealtimes.

PART V

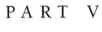

# YOUR THIN
# FOR GOOD
# SUPPLEMENTS

※

# CHAPTER 18

# The Supplement Program

I don't believe any diet can be supported without taking nutritional supplementation. And when I say diet, I mean it in the strictest sense of the word. No matter what we eat or how we eat it, we all need nutritional supplements.

There are a variety of reasons. The most important is that essential nutrients have been depleted from our food supply. This has occurred either through the mineral depletion of the soil in which our plant-based products are grown or in the way we cook (or overcook) our produce. Either way, we deplete nutrients from our foods. And this doesn't even take into account the inordinate amount of pesticides and chemical fertilizers that are placed in the soils of our farms each year.

In the animal products we raise to be eaten, we have destroyed the natural balance of fats and proteins through the feed we use for those animals, the amount of antibiotics farmers are allowed to use by the government, and the growth hormones that are used in order to increase the yield from each animal.

In order to protect our health, I recommend nutritional supplements for everyone, not just for those who will be following my diet program. Whenever you diet, you will naturally be lacking some of the basic nutrients, if only because you cut down on many of the foods you normally eat. These nutrients are essential and must be replaced. Nutrients also help our bodies defend against many of the potential hazards generated by the way the food is delivered to our tables.

I will outline two groups of nutrients, one for dieters, and one for the general population. I recommend that dieters use both groups of nutrients. If you are on any medication, I would advise you to check with your personal physician, or at least with someone who has some knowledge of the benefits of nutritional supplements, before embarking on any nutritional supplementation program I recommend. The last thing in the world I want is for you to harm yourself by following any of the advice in this book. So if at all in doubt, please consult with someone who knows your medical history and also knows something about nutritional supplementation.

# Nutrients for Dieters

Female or male, whatever stage of life you are in, there are some basic nutrients you should be taking. These include a good multivitamin, carnitine, essential fatty acids, chromium, lipoic acid, and coenzyme Q10.

In addition, there are some nutrients that may help with some of the problems you may encounter with dieting. This group includes glutamine, magnesium oxide, taurine, kava-kava, and vitamin $B_6$.

I believe these supplements play a vital role in helping us lose weight and be healthy. But I think it's important that you know about some of the properties of these supplements, so you have some idea why I ask my patients to add them to their diet program. It may also help you to design your own program, without my assistance, should something arise in your diet that might need correction.

## Supplements for All Dieters

### Multivitamin

I recommend that you take 3 to 6 of these per day to ensure that you get many of the minor yet still important players in your daily regimen. A good multivitamin includes manganese, vanadyl sulfate, zinc, niacin, niacinamide, pyridoxal-5 phosphate, vitamin A, and a few others.

### Chromium

This is one of the most valuable supplements that you can take. Despite a short-lived health scare concerning this supplement several years ago (it was reported that chromium could damage your health if taken in a dose equivalent to 6000 times the normal dose), this nutrient has been shown to be a valuable weapon in the arsenal of many dieters. Chromium is a trace mineral that is deficient in a large percentage of the population, primarily because the soil in America has been largely depleted of it.

Chromium is vital to blood sugar regulation and is useful for those who suffer from hypoglycemia or diabetes, as well as anyone who falls between these two extremes of the blood sugar spectrum. It is not possible to get this nutrient from food, as no foods are high in this trace mineral except for brewer's yeast. This is why it must be taken in the form of a nutritional supplement. This mineral has been shown to help increase the body's metabolism and help burn fat. These are two good reasons why I recommend chromium to dieters in a dose of 200 micrograms three to four times per day. Also, you may take an additional 200-microgram dose at any time through the day if you should feel a food craving coming on, because it will help get rid of that craving almost instantly. Chromium is available in the picolinate and the polynicotinate form, either of which is good to take.

### Essential Fatty Acids

These are the omega-3 and omega-6 substances I have been talking about throughout the book. The omega-3 fatty acids are alpha-linolenic acid (ALA), docosahexanoic acid (DHA), and eicosapentanoic acid (EPA). EPA and DHA can be obtained from a good fish oil supplement. There are many brands of oil products that can be found in your local health food store or vitamin store. Look at the ingredients on the label. I generally recommend approximately 1000 mg per day of both DHA and EPA. ALA can be found in flaxseed oil, and I recommend you take 1000 mg per day of this, too, again, in divided doses.

Since we already get so much of the omega-6 fatty acids in our diet, I recommend you take only one additional oil in the form of a supplement: gamma-linolenic acid (GLA) or linoleic acid (LA). It is difficult to synthesize this fatty acid from other sources in your diet, and so it should best be taken in addition to the food you eat each day. GLA can be found in evening primrose oil and borage oil. I recommend either of these capsules, for a daily dose of 1000 mg.

These fatty acids have been shown to help prevent the inflammation of arthritis, decrease blood fat levels, reduce platelet aggregation, and possibly influence blood pressure. Most important, these fatty acids help to regulate the pathways that may cause inflammation in your body. Omega-6 fatty acids, which our diets contain too much of, help to stimulate inflammation, and the omega-3 fatty acids will do the opposite. There is much scientific evidence to support the taking of these on a regular basis. I heartily encourage their use.

### Coenzyme Q10

This nutrient is also known as ubiquinone, because it is ubiquitous, contained in every cell in our bodies. It is an important nutrient not only for the dieter, but for everyone. It has so many good properties. It is a great antioxidant and may help to increase the functioning of the immune system. It is extremely good for cardiac patients, so it is especially helpful in the older male populations, and it has been used to treat such conditions as heart disease, diabetes, and cancer. In some studies, it has been shown to help with congestive heart failure, decreasing angina or chest pain and lowering blood pressure.

So, why do I include this in the essential list for any dieter? Because it is believed that CoQ10 may help your body use its stored fat as energy and fuel for your metabolism. Studies have shown that dieters who took this supplement lost more weight than those who didn't. I recommend this supplement in the range of 100 to 300 mg per day in divided doses, depending on your weight. Those above 200 pounds should take the higher end of this range.

### Lipoic Acid
This supplement is being touted as a great antioxidant and blood sugar regulator. I consider it essential to anyone with blood sugar problems, including diabetes, and any patient with cancer or a history of cancer. It is a powerful protector of the liver, too. I recommend it for dieters because of its effect in blood sugar regulation and because it may help the body convert food into energy in a more efficient way, so that your body does not deposit its food in the form of fat. The dosage I recommend is 100 to 300 mg per day in divided doses with meals.

### Carnitine
This is an amino acid that science has dubbed nonessential. However, I consider it vital to any dieter because it naturally helps your body burn fat to supply its energy needs. It is useful in other conditions such as heart disease and fatigue. I recommend this supplement in the amount of 500 to 1000 mg three times per day, for a total of 1500 to 3000 mg per day. It should be taken before meals or on an empty stomach.

## Supplements to Help with Problems You May Encounter Dieting
This is a grouping of supplements I prescribe for patients to help ease the most common problems they may encounter while they diet. Again, I caution you that although these are very safe to use for just about anyone, you should not take any of these without consulting your physician.

### Glutamine
This is the amino acid that is the most abundant in the body. I give it to my patients to help them primarily with sugar cravings. I have also used it for other addictive behaviors, such as nicotine and alcohol cravings, but I have been most successful using it for the sugar cravings that many dieters experience, especially in the first few days of their new eating plan.

I recommend glutamine in the dose of 500 to 1000 mg three times per day, for a total of 1500 to 3000 mg per day. In addition, you may also take this supplement whenever you feel an urge for something you shouldn't be eating. It should be taken before meals or on an empty stomach to get its full benefit. If you take one or two extra capsules each time you feel a food craving, then wait five minutes, the craving will almost always disappear. This is very helpful for most early-stage dieters.

### Taurine
This is another amino acid that I recommend to my dieters. It has many other uses too, and I have used it to help in other conditions such as high blood pressure, seizure disorders, and edema. That is the main reason why I recommend it to dieters, because it will help you with any fluid retention you may experience. It is especially helpful for women of childbearing age

during the time of the month when they may experience water retention. This supplement may also help in the process of fat metabolism. I recommend a dose of 500 to 1000 mg three times per day for a total of 1500 to 3000 mg, depending on the severity of the water retention. It too should be taken either before meals or on an empty stomach.

### Magnesium Oxide
This valuable nutrient helps with problems of constipation. Many dieters who change the way they have been eating often experience a feeling of being constipated. This is especially likely if you have always followed a high-carbohydrate diet, because there is a lot of bulk in the diet of someone who eats breads and pasta all day. So, you will often experience a change in your bowel movements on a diet higher in protein and lower in carbohydrate. Your stool will be less bulky, and you may experience this as constipation. It is not actual constipation, but simply a diminution in the amount of bulk your body produces in a given day. If this happens, then all you need to do is to take 1 to 3 250-mg tablets of this supplement per day, and the problem should be eliminated. It is not habit-forming.

### Psyllium Husks
This may be taken either in capsule or powder form. Also used for constipation, this supplement acts to bulk up your stool, and it is also non-habit forming. Essentially, this is the active ingredient in many over-the-counter laxative products, but it does not have the sugar that they have.

### Kava-Kava
This is an herbal product that is ideally suited for anyone suffering from anxiety. I put this herb into the dieter's category because many people become anxious when they change their way of eating. Also, many people use food for much more than nutrition, and use it to comfort themselves in times of crisis. I would rather you use this herb, along with the mind-body exercises, and stay away from food.

If you get anxious or upset, for whatever reason, reach for the kava-kava and not the cookie jar. Kava-kava is safe to use, unless you are on some other medication for anxiety, such as Prozac or Valium. Please consult your physician if you are taking any drugs like that before taking this herb, as there may be an interaction. I recommend a dose of 50 to 300 mg per day in divided doses, to be used on an as needed basis.

## General Nutritional Supplements

The nutrients I feel the entire population should be taking include vitamin C, vitamin E, the natural form of beta-carotene, selenium, ginkgo biloba, and folic acid. Women should add calcium, magnesium, vitamin $D_3$, vitamin

K if there is no contraindication, and boron. Older men should add saw palmetto and lycopene. I will discuss these and the reasons why I think you should be taking them by grouping them according to their usefulness.

## Anti-Aging

Who doesn't want to stay youthful forever? This next group of supplements is a short list of those that I feel are the most important for helping you maintain that youthful vigor. Many supplements can be listed here, but I have included only the least controversial of the many that are available and touted as anti-aging.

After the age of twenty-five, brain cells begin to die at the rate of 1 percent per year. After the age of forty, this process may even accelerate, because the brain's reserves of antioxidants and other protective factors start to fall. It is hard to believe that memory loss begins to occur at such an early age, but in fact it does, and we should begin to address this problem sooner rather than later. Antioxidants are an important component to an anti-aging regimen, and they will be discussed in a separate section.

### Acetyl-l-carnitine

This nutrient is believed to help support energy production in the brain cells themselves, helping to prolong their lives. It may help to protect the cells against toxins and other damages. It may even be helpful in the treatment and prevention of Alzheimer's disease. This amino acid also contributes to the stores of other nutrients such as coenzyme Q10 and glutathione. It should be taken before meals or on an empty stomach and the dose is generally 500 mg three times per day for a daily total of 1500 mg.

### Phosphatidyl Serine

This phospholipid plays a crucial role in the building blocks of cell membranes. It is the essential fatty acid for the brain, considering the brain is almost 60 percent fat. It is found in almost all the cells of the body, but in highest concentrations in the membranes of brain cells. This supplement may improve memory, learning, and concentration. It may also help a patient with Alzheimer's disease, and patients with Parkinson's. The recommended daily dose is 100 mg three times per day for a daily total of 300 mg.

### Ginkgo Biloba Extract

This supplement, derived from the ginkgo tree, has been shown to help increase the flow of blood throughout the body, but particularly in the brain, therefore making it valuable for people who have had strokes, Alzheimer's disease, and memory loss. It is an herb, so you should make sure that you are taking a standardized extract. I recommend a dose of 120 to 240 mg per day in divided doses—the smaller amount for the younger person and the larger

amount for the older person. If you are about to undergo a surgical procedure, it is recommended that the use of ginkgo be stopped two weeks prior
as it may interfere with the clotting mechanism of the blood. You should also
consult your physician before taking this if you are taking any other blood-
thinning agents, such as aspirin or Coumadin.

### DHEA (dehydroepiandrosterone)

This has been touted as being able to increase immune function and energy,
give you a better mood and a better memory, and increase your sex drive. It
may do all those things, but I am not ready to recommend it to people I
don't know. The safe thing to say about it is that it may be very valuable in
the fight against aging, and it is something I use in my practice all the time.
The level of it in your bloodstream is easy to measure and absolutely
decreases as we all age. It will also decrease in times of stress as it is produced
primarily by the adrenal glands. If you are interested in this hormone, ask
your doctor to run a DHEA-sulfate blood test and then you can determine
if you need this supplement in your daily nutrient protocol.

### Pregnenolone

This and human growth hormone (HGH) are being touted as anti-aging
miracles. I hesitate to discuss these in this context. If you are interested in
an anti-aging regimen, you need to see a physician who is familiar with
these and other therapies available that may increase your life span, and will
definitely help you to feel better.

## Antioxidants

These play an extremely valuable role in our health. They help to neutral-
ize harmful free radicals in our cells as we age and as we come in contact with
them on a daily basis. There are many antioxidants on the market. I will
mention only the most common ones and the ones that most people should
be taking on a daily basis. This is not meant to be a complete list by any
means; I am only interested in giving you the information any dieter needs.

### Vitamin C

This is one of the most basic nutrients that we need in our lives. We are one
of the few creatures on the planet that cannot synthesize its own vitamin C.
Therefore, we need to take it in the form of a nutritional supplement. Since
the Nobel Prize–winner Linus Pauling championed the use of vitamin C for
everything from the common cold to cancer, there has been a huge running
debate over how much we really should be taking, and frankly, I don't wish
to become part of that debate at this time. I simply want to say that I think
you should be taking 1000 to 3000 mg per day in divided doses. Studies
have shown this vitamin to be effective against the common cold, asthma,

allergies, and macular degeneration, among other conditions, and it is even believed to be effective in helping your body fight cancer by helping strengthen the workings of your immune system. In any case, taking this dosage of vitamin C will certainly not be injurious to your health.

### Vitamin E
This is another "no-brainer" supplement. With all the medical literature (even from the most conventional sources) singing this vitamin's praises, everyone should be taking it. Vitamin E has been shown to help in dealing with heart disease, macular degeneration, menopausal symptoms, cancer, memory problems, and lung diseases, to name a few. There are several versions of this supplement available at your local health food store. I recommend that you look for the natural mixed tocopherols, as that is how the vitamin most closely appears in nature. You should take this in a dose range of 400 to 1200 I.U. per day in divided doses. As this may affect bleeding time, I recommend you take the smaller dose if you are taking anything like aspirin or other blood thinners. Again, you should not be taking supplements just because I recommend them. Each case needs to be individualized, and I encourage you to seek the advice of a knowledgeable physician.

### Beta-Carotene
This vitamin has come under much scrutiny in the past few years. I recommend that you use it in its most natural form to ensure that you receive all the carotenoids. (It is the synthetic beta-carotene that has been shown to cause problems in some medical studies.) Beta-carotene is a powerful antioxidant that has been shown to be helpful in the fight against cancer, heart disease, and eye diseases such as macular degeneration. For those of you who smoke, it is essential that you use the natural and not the synthetic version of this supplement, as the synthetic may cause more harm than good in your particular instance. I recommend 25,000 I.U. per day.

### Selenium
This is a another mineral that is important to our health and that has been depleted from our soil. Therefore, it must be taken in the form of a nutritional supplement to achieve its benefit. Selenium has been shown to fight against cancer, especially prostate cancer. I recommend a dose of 50 to 200 micrograms per day, in divided doses.

## Keeping Your Heart Healthy

Since heart disease is the single largest killer of Americans, causing one in five deaths, it is a good idea to take something that may protect your heart. The essential things that you need for heart health are the supplements that can help to lower your cholesterol, counteract the free radical effect, and help increase oxygen flow to the vessels around your heart. Again, there are numerous supplements I can mention here. The most important ones are the antioxidants that have previously been described, coenzyme Q10, the essential fatty acids, and magnesium.

## Magnesium

This is an extremely valuable mineral that has been shown to help in many of the most common health problems today, most notably high blood pressure, asthma, and migraine headaches. I mention this mineral as a "must-have" for women because it helps your body absorb the necessary calcium it needs to protect against bone loss and osteoporosis. It is also a must for men to use because of the beneficial effects it may have on the heart. It has been shown to be able to increase the delivery of oxygen to the heart and relax the peripheral blood vessels, leading to a lowering of blood pressure. It has also been shown to be helpful in cardiac arrhythmias such as atrial fibrillation, the most common. It has even been shown to be effective for migraine headaches.

Again, there are many forms available from your local health food store. The forms I like the best are orotate and taurate. I recommend 600 to 750 mg of either form per day in divided doses along with your calcium (covered later). Too much magnesium may cause diarrhea in some people. If this happens to you, decrease the amount of magnesium you take per day and slowly build the dose back up to the optimum level.

## Pantethine

This is the most important supplement you can take to help control your cholesterol. This member of the B vitamin family is directly involved in the metabolism of all the food components, and is also the basis for the production of many important players in our body, such as hemoglobin and the sex hormones, to name a few. It may also help encourage the body to produce enzymes that help break down fats—an important component to heart health—and lower triglyceride and cholesterol levels. I recommend a dose of 150 mg three times each day.

## Folic Acid

This is another nutritional supplement that has been getting a lot of positive press lately, and for very good reason. It is probably the vitamin all of us need most because our food supply has been depleted of this as a result of food processing. Only recently has it started to be added to processed food products. Two of the most important things folic acid has been shown to do include decreasing the incidence of birth defects and decreasing your homocysteine level (a potent indicator of heart disease). It also has a positive estrogenic effect in very high doses and may be important to women not only in their childbearing years but for many years after that. This is a prescription supplement in large doses, but you can get it over the counter in the form of 800-microgram tablets. I would recommend that you take two of these per day.

## Eye Health

The two leading problems of failing eyesight, macular degeneration and cataracts, may be helped by simply taking some nutritional supplements. The aim is to decrease the effect of free radical formation. Since sunlight causes a great many of these free radicals to form, and the eye directly takes in the light we need to see, antioxidants are the key players in the fight for good eye health. Ginkgo biloba extract and bilberry may also play a role in eye protection.

### Lutein and Zeaxanthin

These bioflavonoids from the carotenoid family are two important players in the quest for good eye health. They help filter the damaging blue rays of the sun before they can cause damage to the macula. These should be taken in the amount of 10,000 I.U. three times per day, for a daily total of 30,000 I.U.

# Supplements Specific for Women

As in many other aspects of our lives, men and women differ in the nutritional supplements they require. For this reason, I would like to recommend the following supplements for the women reading this book. I do this because these may aid in the two most common conditions that affect women as they age: osteoporosis/osteoarthritis and menopause.

## Osteoporosis and Osteoarthritis

### Calcium

After folic acid, calcium is the nutritional supplement women need most, regardless of their age. This is a mineral that helps keep your bones healthy, but it is also vital to the body for many other functions. It has been shown to be helpful in controlling high blood pressure, building strong teeth, and even aiding against insomnia, colon cancer, and premenstrual syndrome. There are many forms of calcium available on the market today. In my own practice, I have found the aspartate and the citrate forms to be the most readily absorbed and most easily tolerated. Regardless of the form of calcium you choose, you need to take 1200 to 1500 mg per day in divided doses. This supplementation should be started as early as the teenage years. In order for calcium to be properly absorbed by the body, it needs the help of magnesium, as I've previously described, and it needs help in the form of the two nutritional supplements I'll mention next.

### Vitamin D$_3$

This is an important player because it will help your body absorb the necessary calcium. Most of us do not get the amount of light our bodies need to synthesize this vitamin. And, the darker your skin tone, the harder it is for your body to do this by itself. I recommend you take 400 I.U. per day in the months of April through October and 800 I.U. per day in divided doses in the months of November through March. The opposite is true if you are reading this book in the Southern Hemisphere.

### Vitamin K

This vitamin is important for the prevention of osteoporosis. Without it, our bodies cannot form osteocalcin, which is a necessary component of new bone growth. Recent studies have shown this vitamin to be extremely beneficial, yet it should be taken with caution and only under the guidance of a physician because it affects your body's coagulation process. This means that if you are taking any blood thinners, such as aspirin, Coumadin, or one of the newer agents on the market, you would need to regulate the dosage. I recommend that only immediate postmenopausal women begin this supplement and take only 100 micrograms per day.

### Boron

I recommend this for women because it will help keep their bones healthy. Studies have shown this mineral to be able to decrease the urinary loss of calcium, a valuable thing in anyone concerned with osteoporosis. I recommend a dose of 3 mg per day. As this may have some influence on estrogen, women with a history of a hormonally related cancer, such as breast or ovarian cancer, should consult their physicians before taking this supplement.

### Glucosamine Sulfate

This is especially helpful in the treatment of arthritis, and applies to both women and men. The body manufactures its own supply of glucosamine, which aids in the buildup of cartilage. But as we age, the body is unable to continue to produce as much as we need, and the joints begin to deteriorate. I recommend a dose of 1000 mg three times a day for a daily total of 3000 mg.

## Menopause

The important components to a good nutritional supplement program for anyone in the menopausal time of life would include soy, black cohosh, and red clover.

### Red Clover

This contains phytoestrogens, which may help regulate hormone levels and alleviate those annoying hot flashes. I recommend a dose of 45 mg of a standardized extract three times per day.

### Black Cohosh

This has been studied throughout Europe with good results. Again, it is a phytoestrogen, which means that it contains small amounts of an estrogenic substance. It may be able to help balance the hormonal disturbances that make menopause so uncomfortable. I recommend a dose of 15 mg three times per day.

# Supplements for Men

I have only four additional supplements to add to your repertoire at this point, and these supplements are recommended only for men over forty. They have to do with sexual function and sexual organ health.

### Saw Palmetto

This herb has been shown to be helpful for your prostate. It has been shown to alleviate many of the symptoms of an enlarged prostate (known as benign prostatic hypertrophy, or BPH) such as urinary frequency, urinary urgency, and nocturia (nighttime urination) even better than the prescription medications used to treat this condition. I feel you should take this supplement even if you are not experiencing any of the symptoms yet. I use it as a preventative measure with most of my male patients, and I recommend a dose of 160 mg three times per day.

### Lycopene

This is a food substance from the tomato that has been found to help against prostate cancer. Dietarily it is better obtained through cooked tomato products rather than raw. There is no standardized extract, so I would recommend 3 capsules per day in divided doses.

### L-arginine

This is another important amino acid. Your body will convert L-arginine to nitric oxide, which is then absorbed by the smooth muscle cells that line your arteries. This will increase blood flow and can help men who have trouble with impotence. I have used this with my patients with some success instead of Viagra. It also plays the same role in the heart and may be used for patients with angina or chest pain. The dose is 3 grams three times per day, before meals or on an empty stomach, for a daily dose of 9 grams.

### Choline

This is the raw material your body uses to send nerve impulses throughout the body. It is converted into acetylcholine in the body, and when taken in conjunction with vitamin $B_5$, the necessary material to aid in this conversion, it may increase sexual stimulation. This will also apply to the women in the audience, so you may want to experiment with your partner.

However, once again I caution you always to check with a knowledge-able physician before taking any of the supplements discussed in this chapter, especially if you are on any other medication for the same or other problems.

There are many reasons to take nutritional supplements. I have only begun to scratch the surface of how valuable they are in the treatment of many of the most common illnesses we face today. It is possible to follow the Thin For Good diet without taking even a single vitamin supplement and still lose weight. But my experience has shown it will be easier and more beneficial if you use the supplements I have recommended.

The decision on nutritional supplementation is entirely up to you.

PART VI

ENHANCING

THIN FOR GOOD

# CHAPTER 19

# Move It

Let's face it, you knew I had to discuss exercise at some point in this book. There are so many excuses for not exercising that it is almost comical: "The weather's bad," "I have a cold," "I'm too tired," "Who's going to watch the kids?" They all tell me the same thing. No matter how you say it, you just hate to exercise. However, I would bet that my daily doses of mind-body medicine can help you overcome your fears or anxieties about exercise, too.

You're certainly not alone in disliking exercise. More than 60 percent of all North Americans get little or no exercise. But don't comfort yourself by saying, "Well, I'm not alone." Because, if you give it some thought, you'll realize that 60 percent is also the percentage of Americans who are overweight.

Now for the good news, or at least news that may make you feel better about the whole idea of exercising. The American College of Sports Medicine recently revised its guidelines for exercise to maintain fitness as well as to help in weight control.

Instead of the traditional activities we have all come to associate with physical fitness, such as jogging, aerobics, and the like, the experts are now telling us that all we have to do is to incorporate more movement into our daily routine. Sounds easy, doesn't it? Well, it is, and it's something I have been encouraging my patients to do for years. Nevertheless, most of us find even that too difficult to do.

## What Can Exercise Really Do for You?

Studies have shown that vigorous, sustained exercise can help fight heart disease, hypertension, diabetes, stroke, and osteoporosis. Yet, fewer than one-fifth of us engage in regular physical activity of this kind, defined as any activity that increases your heart rate to at least 85 percent of the maximum predicted at least four times per week for at least 20 minutes. (See page 216 to determine your maximum heart rate.) Also, several researchers have suggested that becoming more fit can take twenty years off a person's chronological age by delaying the onset of limitations that affect people that are not physically fit.

Since this is primarily a diet book, I should point out that the best thing exercise can do for you is to help you shed some weight by increasing your basal metabolic rate. But there's more. Exercise may also help prevent back pain by improving the back's strength, flexibility, and endurance. And here's an extra benefit: exercise has been shown to increase self-esteem and energy, improve your mood and your love life, and decrease stress. All these things can also help you stay on your new diet regimen. Therefore, exercise helps not only in boosting your metabolism and increasing your resting muscle mass, but in psychological ways as well.

Since I have talked about insulin and its many effects on the body throughout this book, I should add here that anything that contributes to weight loss will help to maintain better control of your insulin level. Overweight individuals are frequently insulin resistant. Exercise can help you lose weight and help you become less insulin resistant by clearing up the underlying cause—obesity.

## The New Guidelines

For the first time, the new exercise guidelines include a recommendation for flexibility training in addition to aerobic and strength training. Flexibility simply means that stretching should be incorporated into your fitness program, and it is recommended that you do this three days per week. As for the aerobic guidelines, it is recommended that these be performed three to five days per week for 20 to 60 minutes each time, at an intensity that raises your heart rate to 55 to 90 percent of maximum. One of these sessions may be replaced by two to six 10-minute periods of aerobic activity throughout the day.

It is important to know how to test your heart rate so that you can follow these recommendations, if you so choose. Simply turn one hand palm up and place the first two fingers of the opposite hand on the thumb side of your wrist, and you will feel your pulse. You may have to move your fingers a little bit to find the right spot, as it is slightly different in everyone, and you should not apply too much pressure. Then just count the beats for one minute and that is your pulse rate.

The two numbers you want to know are your resting pulse rate and your maximum pulse rate. The resting pulse rate is easy, because that will be the number you get when you are not doing any physical activity, such as now, while you are reading this book. Unless you have a physical malady or are taking certain medications, the slower your resting heart rate, the better shape you are in.

The maximum projected heart rate is a function of age, not fitness. The standard formula is: 220 minus your age equals what your maximum heart rate should be. You are generally shooting for 85 percent of your maximum heart rate when you are exercising. For example, if you are fifty years old, your maximum predicted heart rate would be $220 - 50 = 170$; 85 percent of $170 = 147$. This should be the fastest your heart should beat during aerobic exercises. This is sometimes referred to as target heart rate.

The recommendations for resistance training are based on the amount of time, the degree of training, and how suitable it is for the majority of adults. Recommendations include one set of 8 to 10 exercises that work the major muscle groups two to three days each week.

## The Latest Studies

Now at last, something we can all live with: A recently published study, conducted under the direction of Dr. Andrea Dunn of the Cooper Institute for Aerobic Research in Dallas, showed that in previously sedentary (yes, that's most of you) healthy adults, a lifestyle physical activity intervention is as effective as a structured exercise program in improving physical activity, cardio-respiratory fitness, and blood pressure.

This means that, for the first time, someone has shown that by increasing the activities you do in your daily life, you will get some positive health impacts. You do not have to become a gym junkie to achieve health benefits. This is something many of us can live with, since we do most of these activities on a daily basis anyway.

## How to Get Started

By using everyday events, you can tailor physical activity uniquely to your lifestyle. If you have not been physically active, start slowly and gradually increase the time and pace of your activity. Choose an activity you enjoy, or something that needs to get done anyway, and do it at a convenient time. Choose a variety of different activities to avoid getting bored. Try to exercise regularly. This means you should aim for at least 20 minutes three times each week. Now, it may take you six months or more to reach that level of activity, but that's perfectly all right. Just do something.

Like dieting, exercise is something that should remain with you for the rest of your life, and therefore it is not a race against time to get to the maximum level. Get your family—especially your children, if you have any—involved, too. If you are more physically active, chances are your children will be too, and then they will most likely stay active as adults.

Entire families exercising together is the real key to success. I use the term family very loosely. This may be friends, relatives, neighbors, co-workers or anyone that is willing to commit to exercising together. It makes exercise more enjoyable, more of an activity, and the minutes seem to fly by much more quickly when you exercise with someone else—at least they do for me.

# The Lifestyle Activities

Lifestyle activities or everyday events are those things you would normally do in the course of a day, such as taking a brisk walk around the block, raking leaves, using the stairs instead of the elevator, polishing furniture, vacuuming the house, playing with the kids in the park, parking at the far end of the parking lot, washing dishes, carrying groceries, pushing a cart while grocery shopping, washing the car, walking the dog, gardening—even having sex.

The first ever Surgeon General's report on Physical Activity and Health, released in July 1996, concluded that regular, moderate physical activity can substantially reduce the risk of developing or dying from heart disease, diabetes, colon cancer, or high blood pressure. This report defined moderate physical activity as that which expends 150 calories per day, or 1000 calories per week. This is pretty easy to attain when you increase your level of lifestyle activities and include such things as:

- walking briskly for 30 minutes
- swimming laps for 20 minutes
- washing and waxing a car for 45 minutes
- pushing a stroller 1½ miles in 30 minutes
- playing volleyball for 45 minutes
- playing touch football for 30 to 45 minutes
- walking on a treadmill for a mile in 20 minutes
- shooting baskets for 20 minutes
- bicycling 5 miles in 30 minutes
- fast dancing for 30 minutes
- doing water aerobics for 30 minutes
- playing a game of basketball or soccer for 15 to 20 minutes
- bicycling 4 miles in 15 minutes
- jumping rope for 15 minutes
- running 1½ miles in 15 minutes
- stair walking for 15 minutes
- playing baseball for 45 minutes

These lifestyle activities offer similar health benefits and can be a suitable alternative to more vigorous exercise for people who are not able or who don't like to perform vigorous exercise. I heartily encourage you to participate in some level of exercise. Look for ways to make it fun and to incorporate it into your daily life. If you don't do that, then it will always be relegated to an "if I have the time for that" sort of thing. Just do something extra each day. Walk to the store, walk to get lunch, walk an extra lap around the mall without stopping, walk the dog an extra block in each direction, pick up the kids from school without the car. There are so many ways to do this without even feeling that you have done something.

## Sex-Rated Activities

What could be better than combining two activities and getting benefits from both? This can help bring couples closer together, and, for older couples, it can help maintain the intimacy that sometimes gets lost as couples age together and start to take one another for granted. Here are some fun activities that also burn calories.

- Kissing for 30 minutes = 50 calories
- Making out for 30 minutes = 100 calories
- Intercourse for 30 minutes (to guys this may seem impossible) = 225 calories
- Massage for 30 minutes = 75 calories
- Vigorous foreplay for 30 minutes = 150 calories

Sort of makes you think twice about "not tonight dear, I have a headache," doesn't it? Just think, if you did this and increased your everyday activities, how much better shape you and your partner would be in.

## Be Careful

If done properly, exercise is safe for almost everyone. If you are pregnant (in which case you should not be following my weight loss diet); if you are taking any heart medication, especially for high blood pressure; or if you have any medical condition, such as arthritis, that may be aggravated by exercise—consult your doctor about what level of activity and what types of activity are acceptable for you.

## Setting Goals

It is important to set realistic goals for yourself. Don't kid yourself into thinking that you will be able to start a new diet, start exercising, and stop smoking all on the same day. It's probable that you will fail when you set such unrealistic expectations for yourself. I think the reason many people decide to do all those things at once is so that they will fail with at least one of the things and then use that as an excuse to stop the others.

Remember, some activity is better than none at all, no matter at what level you are able to perform. Don't think of yourself as a failure simply because you can't run that marathon. Don't think of yourself as a failure even if you don't do any exercise at all. Just do the best you can, and you'll get healthier simply by trying and succeeding at a small fraction of what I have discussed. If you are afraid of the word exercise, then increasing your lifestyle activities is the thing for you. Have fun with exercise if you can, because that is the only way you are ever going to be able to keep at it.

CHAPTER 20

# Overcoming Special Weight Loss Difficulties

This chapter is about the five most common reasons why some people may have difficulty losing weight on this or any other diet. In my years of clinical practice, I have found these reasons, more than any other, to be the cause of most of the problems that my patients experienced. I am not going to discuss the most obvious reason, which is cheating or not following the instructions, because in that case the reason for your failure to lose weight is quite clear.

These are the problems I look for when I have determined that a patient has been following my program to the letter and I can find no other reason for their lack of progress.

## The Yeast Situation

What follows is information that you'll probably never get from your conventionally oriented physician because he or she likely doesn't believe that the problem I'm going to describe even exists. Nevertheless, this condition affects a large percentage of the population. If you are one of those who suffers from this condition, the restrictions I will discuss in this chapter relate to you.

The yeast I refer to is called *Candida albicans*, a naturally occurring fungus that lives in our digestive tract. The balance between good and bad bacteria in our digestive tract becomes destroyed when we take antibiotics, birth control pills, steroids (such as prednisone), and when we are pregnant or have diabetes. These circumstances will cause the yeast in our body to overgrow, sacrificing the good bacteria.

### Do I Have Yeast?

There are many symptoms that can indicate a yeast infection, or more specifically a yeast overgrowth. Some of the most common are gastrointestinal problems such as bowel irregularities, bloating, gas, indigestion, or heartburn. Another set of symptoms that may be attributable to yeast overgrowth include classic allergy symptoms, such as asthma, hives, runny nose, sinus problems, acne, eczema, brain fog, lightheadedness, and even attention deficit, to name a few. Many of my female patients think they could never have a yeast problem because they have never had a vaginal yeast infection; male patients think this condition is only for women. *Candida* is a naturally occurring organism in all of our bodies. Therefore, any one of us can be bothered by these symptoms.

## Controlling Yeast

If you are experiencing any of these symptoms or have had them in the not-too-distant past, or have chronically been on the medications listed above, and you are having difficulty losing weight, I would recommend that you add a yeast restriction to your diet. The most therapeutic way of controlling yeast is to adjust your diet, take certain nutritional supplements that will help your gut restore the balance of the good bacteria, and do something that may help kill the yeast itself. The ultimate aim of the treatment is to restore the body's own natural balance to what it should be.

One of the primary things you need to eliminate from your diet to control yeast is sugar, which is what you are already doing by following this diet. You also must eliminate yeast products or anything that contains yeast. This includes everything that rises, like breads and bagels, something else you are already doing if you are on my diet program.

Another category of foods to eliminate is fruit because of the sugar it contains. By the same token, you need to eliminate sweet potatoes, corn, carrots, beets, peas, and lima beans. If you suffer from this yeast condition you must eliminate cheese of any kind, but especially the hard or aged cheeses. The soft cheeses are not fermented, but they do contain a small amount of sugar so it's best to avoid these, too.

Mushrooms, because they are a type of fungus, must also be avoided, as should fermented food of any kind, which includes vinegar, soy sauce, sauerkraut, sour cream, mayonnaise, and mustard.

The following two tables should better help you figure out which foods to avoid and which you may enjoy.

### Foods to Be Avoided on a Yeast-Free Diet

| | | |
|---|---|---|
| alcoholic beverages | catsup | dried roasted nuts |
| all foods containing sugar | cereals with sugar | fermented beverages |
| | cheese | flour |
| barbecue sauce | cookies | frozen or canned citrus fruits and juices |
| biscuits | cottage cheese | |
| breads | crackers | |
| buttermilk | dried and cured foods | hamburger and hot dog buns |
| candy | dried fruits | |

horseradish
mayonnaise
milk
mushrooms
pastries
pickles
pretzels

root beer
rolls
sauerkraut
smoked foods
sour cream
soy sauce

store-bought salad
    dressings
teas
tomato sauce
truffles
vinegar

---

Note: Milk is not allowed on a yeast-free diet because of the sugar in the milk.

Now that we know all the things you can't eat, here are some of the foods that are permitted, depending on which phase of the Thin For Good diet program you are in.

### Foods That Can Be Eaten on a Yeast-Free Diet

| Whole Grains | Breads | Cereals | Whole Grain Pastas |
|---|---|---|---|
| rice—short, medium, and long (brown preferable, but white may be used) cracked wheat bulgur wheat couscous millet oats barley buckwheat groats (kasha) quinoa amaranth | yeast-free breads like sourdough, rye, essene, spelt, kamut, and multi-grain corn tortillas chapatis (made from wheat) | *hot cereals:* wheat, oat, rice, mixed grain cereals  *cold cereals:* shredded wheat puffed wheat puffed millet puffed corn puffed rice puffed kasha | whole wheat pasta (also called udon) artichoke pasta corn pasta (wheat-free) rice pasta (wheat-free) buckwheat pasta (also called soba) |

A yeast-restricted diet does not last forever, but to truly rid yourself of a yeast problem, you must adhere to these restrictions for at least three months if you do it to the letter, and up to six to nine months if you cheat. Once you have completed the three to nine months of the yeast restrictions, then you have to slowly transition yourself back to eating foods that contain yeast. The first products I would add are the mustard, mayonnaise, and other foods that contain vinegar. After that, you may want to add the soft cheeses, and then you may add the hard cheeses. The last things you should add are the breads with yeast. In your local health-food store, you can find many breads made without yeast.

Keep in mind that you have gone without these foods for several months by this point, so there is no reason to rush back into having them. If any of the original symptoms reappear once you start incorporating these foods back into your diet, then you must decrease the food that caused the symptom and increase the foods with yeast more slowly into your diet. If yeast was the reason you were unable to lose weight on the original initiation phase, this will more than likely have corrected the problem and the weight loss should now be occurring.

## Yeast-Fighting Supplements

There are several supplements I use to help control yeast problems in my patients. They are garlic, caprylic acid, grapefruit seed extract, and the substances known as probiotics. The former supplements are used to help your body to kill the yeast cell itself. Probiotics are essentially the opposite of antibiotics, as they replenish your gut with the good flora that antibiotics destroy or have destroyed in the past. These include *Lactobacillus acidophilus*, *Lactobacillus bulgaricus*, and *Bifidobacterium bifidum*.

To sum up, if you want to avoid a re-infection of the yeast, you should:

- Avoid antibiotics.
- If you require antibiotics, make sure you replace the beneficial bacteria by using probiotics, such as acidophilus and bifidus, during the entire time you are on the antibiotic and then for ten days after the antibiotic course has been completed.
- Follow a yeast-free diet.
- Avoid sugar.

# Thyroid Problems

This is often underdiagnosed in the general population. The primary reason is that the biochemical tests that are available to test for thyroid problems are inadequate and because routine screening is often not done because of cost-cutting. Traditional tests are able to measure your thyroid hormone and your thyroid-stimulating hormone, but they are unable to measure how your body is able to process these hormones. Your blood tests may be perfectly normal, but the hormones may not be functioning as they were intended to do.

Also, hypothyroidism—or a slow or underactive thyroid—is more common than was formerly believed. The medical community is now calling for anyone over the age of fifty to be screened for this condition. The screening test for this checks levels of TSH, or thyroid-stimulating hormone. If this is too high, then you have hypothyroidism. Unfortunately, using this definition, many of the subtle cases are missed.

### How Do I Know If I Have a Thyroid Problem?

Do you feel more fatigued than you should? Is your hair thinning? Are your bowel movements irregular? Do your fingernails crack or are they brittle? Do you have high cholesterol? Do you experience brain fog? Are you having difficulty losing weight? There are probably close to a hundred symptoms on this list, far too many to mention here. However, these are the most classic symptoms and the ones I use to determine if my patient has a low thyroid problem.

Another test that I use—something that you can do easily at home—is to rub a small square of colored iodine somewhere on your skin. I usually recommend using the inner thigh or the upper arm, as these two spots are generally hidden by clothing. Try to place this spot in an area you will not be washing throughout the day to ensure an accurate measurement. If that spot takes less than 24 hours to disappear, then you have a thyroid that is not functioning up to par.

The third thing I look for are basal body temperatures. I ask my patients to take their temperature with a glass bulb thermometer, not a digital one, four times a day, once before each meal and at bedtime, for four days in a row. If the average temperature is under 98 degrees, then I would consider the patient to have an underactive thyroid. This is another quick-and-easy test you can do at home to see if that is the reason you may be having difficulty with weight loss.

### Correcting the Problem

If one of my patients were to experience any problems like this, I would seriously consider putting them on a low-dose, all-natural thyroid medication, especially if he or she is having difficulty losing weight. If this sounds like you, I encourage you to see your regular physician and ask for a thyroid blood test.

The only real way to treat this condition is to take a natural thyroid extract that needs to be prescribed by a physician. Other natural things that you can take without a prescription include kelp and magnesium.

# Food Allergies

Food allergies constitute another very common reason some people may have difficulty losing weight. Most food allergies are really food sensitivities. By that, I mean that it is not a true allergy, which would cause an obvious reaction, such as hives or difficulty breathing. Rather, a food sensitivity means your body has a minor difficulty processing a particular food. You may get a slight runny nose, slight headache, fatigue, brain fog, or even indigestion—nothing major. And it is probably often overlooked because it is nothing that you can quite put your finger on. Yet it can play a significant role in slowing down your weight loss process. However, food sensitivities may cause some pretty serious symptoms, too, such as acne, eczema, insomnia, sinus problems, diarrhea, and even depression.

### How Do I Know If I Have Food Allergies?

In my practice, I test almost everyone for these food sensitivities either through a cytotoxic food test or through any one of a number of tests that many different companies provide. These tests, which are unlike the food allergy tests that you would receive from your conventional physician, often provide me with the information I need to truly build a specific diet plan for my patients. The most common foods to which people are sensitive are corn, wheat, and other grains; yeast or molds; coffee, pepper, and tomato.

### Correcting the Problem

Since you will not have the benefit of these tests, you can try to eliminate certain foods. First, keep a food diary and write down any symptoms you feel, no matter how subtle they may be. After a week, you should have a good idea of which foods may be giving you trouble. Then, you only need to eliminate those foods, and see if it makes any difference in your weight loss. You may also try eliminating the foods I mentioned above, as they are the most common foods people are sensitive to. You may also want to try the following tips:

- Resist overeating.
- Don't eat too much of the same food at any one sitting.
- Add variety to your diet.

## Hormonal Imbalances

Hormonal imbalances are especially common in women, although they may occur in men, too. The hormones that I look for are DHEA, as I have previously described, and, of course, the sex hormones. As I have explained in previous chapters, losing weight is especially difficult for women about to undergo menopause or those who are currently in menopause. These issues need to be addressed and discussed with your personal physician. You may need to change your medication or you may need certain supplements to help this process along. For more information, please refer to the section on supplements for menopause and aging. Trying some of the supplements I have mentioned in these sections may help to move your weight loss along if you find yourself getting stuck.

## Prescription Drugs

Prescription drugs are an important area to consider if you find you are having difficulty losing weight. In no way do I mean that you should get off the drugs that have been prescribed for you. If you do that, you are doing so at your own risk. If you have any doubts, you should speak with your personal physician. But in my clinical practice, I have found certain drugs cause resistance to weight loss. These include the heart medications such as beta blockers; the antidepressant drugs such as Prozac, Paxil, and others like them; hormone replacement therapy, such as Premarin and Provera; oral hypoglycemics that diabetics take, especially if they are too tightly controlled.

These are the drugs I have found to be the most troublesome to my patients who desire weight loss. This is not to say that it is impossible to lose weight while taking those medications, but some prescription medications may be potential roadblocks in your quest to lose weight. I am sure that if you are taking any of these drugs, it is for very specific reasons and you should not stop your medication without first consulting your physician.

These are the top five reasons I have found why people have difficulty with my diet program. This doesn't mean you should not even attempt this plan if one of these applies to you. I only offer this advice so that you get as complete a picture as possible and don't get discouraged. Remember, no excuses!

✖

# Additional Mind-Body Exercises

Here are many more mind-body medicines I have used with my patients in their quest to lose weight and maintain their weight once it is gone. I recommend you use all these and ponder the meaning they may have in your life. There are many more days ahead of you in which you will be thin. You will need as much help as you can get. I should know—I rely on these doses on a daily basis.

1. Use the power of your mind to your advantage.
2. Know you will succeed.
3. Be happy with any weight loss.
4. Be committed to the program.
5. Have no expectations.
6. You have the power to make this fun.
7. Don't let anyone defeat you.
8. Tap into the positive energy of the universe.
9. Speak about the thinner you.
10. Alert others to your new nutritional lifestyle program.
11. You are only as successful as you allow yourself to be.
12. Don't sabotage yourself.
13. Be the "I" in diet.
14. You are in control of what you eat.
15. Commitment is not a momentary thing.
16. Rid the house of the food you can't eat.
17. Create the future.
18. Turn all the negatives into positives.
19. Learn something from this experience.
20. Know you will not cheat.
21. Be happy with your health gains.
22. Commit to weight loss.
23. Expectations lead to disappointment.
24. Disappointment leads to failure.

25. You have the power to make this successful.
26. You control what is negative about your life.
27. Dieting is not boring.
28. Be powerful.
29. Don't be controlled by your ego.
30. Acknowledge your frustration.
31. Don't make losing weight any more than it is.
32. It's okay to not "look good" all the time.
33. Commit to the mind-body doses.
34. You are in control of what you don't eat.
35. Food does not call out your name.
36. Don't let that wedding defeat you.
37. Love your meals.
38. Use your mind-body index cards when you have a craving.
39. You have the power to make this miserable—don't!
40. Speak about the healthier you.
41. Know what thin looks like.
42. Be confident in your success.
43. Take full responsibility for being overweight or unhealthy.
44. Learn this new program for life.
45. Shop for your new foods and walk around the store an extra time for good luck.
46. Acknowledge your cravings, but don't give in to them.
47. Your life depends on your health—act as if it does.
48. Commit to the 30-day initiation phase.
49. This diet is about you and no one else.
50. Create a new recipe today.
51. Know you can make it through another day.
52. Be comfortable with the new you.
53. Speak the future.
54. Patience holds the key to success.
55. Prepare others for the new you.
56. Don't allow others to sabotage your success by their thoughts.
57. Love your snacks.
58. Don't let what others say mean more to you than your commitment.
59. Boredom is not an excuse to cheat.
60. Acknowledge your fear of success.
61. Find new places to eat out.
62. Weighing yourself once per week is sufficient.
63. Plan a week's menus.
64. Commit to the forever phase.
65. Go on a diet because you want to.

66. Sex-related activities burn calories, too.
67. The time to overcome your overweight mindset is now.
68. Enlist the help of those around you.
69. Think yourself thin.
70. Stay focused.
71. Thinking this is easy is just as easy as thinking this is hard.
72. Your consciousness has no limitations.
73. Know that you will have negative thoughts.
74. Don't make getting healthier any more than what it is.
75. Start a list of your lifestyle activities and see where they can be increased.
76. Mind-body doses are mandatory.
77. Don't put yourself into negative dieting situations.
78. Commit to exercise.
79. Cheating and commitment can't exist in the same game plan.
80. Acknowledge your fear of failure.
81. Boredom is not an excuse to quit.
82. Know that your craving will go away.
83. Don't let that bar mitzvah defeat you.
84. Thrive on the fear of the unknown.
85. Don't lose sight of the bigger picture.
86. Encourage help from those around you by sticking to your ideals.
87. Don't let others sabotage your success by their activities.
88. Have you forgotten you are in control?
89. Drink enough water.
90. Don't hold your success over anyone's head.
91. Don't think about dinner today.
92. This may hurt at times.
93. Start a lifestyle activity group.
94. Be happy with those five pounds.
95. Plan a party around your new nutritional lifestyle program.
96. Go to a health-food store.
97. Ignore all the negative energy around you.
98. Understand that even irrational thoughts can lead you astray.
99. Use your mind-body index cards at home.
100. Think like a thin person.
101. Exercise can give you a better sex life.
102. Have a conversation with your saboteurs.
103. No excuses.
104. Don't blame your failure on anyone but yourself.
105. Turn negative energy into positive by continuing on your road to thinness no matter what.
106. Know you may always be that overweight person—inside.

107. Anger at your _____ does not allow you to cheat.
108. Weight loss is not a competitive sport.
109. Know your weight loss will continue if you are committed.
110. Learn your food labels.
111. There will always be another brownie (or _____).
112. Put your mind to this.
113. Use your mind-body index cards at work.
114. You created the boredom, now un-create it.
115. Limit your time with those who do not support your endeavors.
116. Know there are no limitations to your success.
117. Do thin people dream about chocolate?
118. Make a list of all the positive things you've done since starting the Thin For Good diet.
119. Know the food demons may always be with you.
120. Commit to what you say.
121. Success is within your reach—go for it!
122. Acknowledge that you may always desire the wrong foods—just don't eat them.
123. Teach your kids how to read food labels.
124. Visualize thinness.
125. Is it that hard to find five minutes to exercise each day?
126. Be aware of where the pitfalls lie and avoid them.
127. Use your mind-body index cards in the car.
128. Have fun.
129. Embrace joy.
130. Share your success.
131. One day at a time.

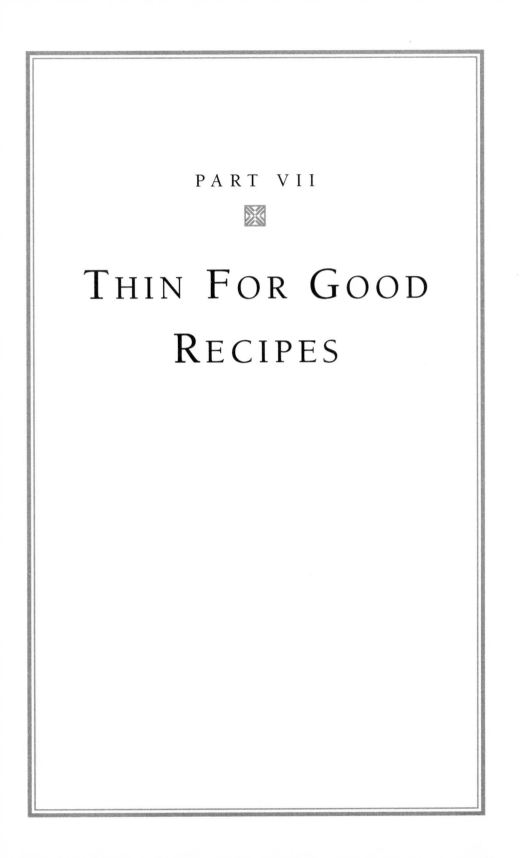

PART VII

THIN FOR GOOD

RECIPES

# CHAPTER 22

# The Recipes

## ⊠ BREAKFAST SELECTIONS ⊠

### Ham 'n Eggs   SERVES 2

1 large slice ham (check that it is not sugar cured)
8 blanched fresh asparagus spears
1 ounce grated cheddar cheese
1 ounce grated natural Swiss cheese
2 poached eggs
2 tablespoons minced parsley

Preheat broiler. Slice the ham on the bias into 3-inch-long strips. Arrange the strips in the bottoms of two gratin dishes or ramekins. Place four asparagus spears over the ham in each dish. Sprinkle on the grated cheese. Place the dishes under the broiler until the cheese bubbles. Remove from the oven and top each dish with a poached egg. Garnish with the minced parsley divided equally.

### Sunday Special Treat   SERVES 6
#### (Ricotta Pancakes with Smoked Salmon)

1 15-ounce container ricotta cheese
4 eggs
⅓ cup whole grain soy flour
2 tablespoons melted butter
1 teaspoon vanilla extract
1 cup sour cream
3 ounces smoked salmon, cut into ¼-inch strips (optional)

Preheat oven to 250°.

Put the ricotta into the bowl of a food processor or blender and whirl until smooth. Add the eggs, one at a time, then add the flour, the melted butter, and the vanilla. Blend until smooth.

Using a gravy ladle, spoon five 2-inch pancakes into a nonstick skillet (if you do not have a nonstick skillet, use a minimal amount of butter to coat the pan), and cook until golden. Turn once and remove to an oven-safe plate. Use remaining batter in the same fashion, keeping each batch warm in the oven. The batter will make 30 pancakes.

Place 5 pancakes on each plate, top with ¼-cup sour cream and smoked salmon if desired.

## *Corned Beef Hash*　SERVES 4

3　pounds corned beef
1　cup shredded cabbage
1　small dill pickle

4　poached eggs
white pepper
2　tablespoons butter

*Garnishes:*
1 tomato, thinly sliced

4 ounces cheddar cheese, grated

Place the corned beef in a large stockpot and cover with water. Cook, covered, for 3 hours. At the end of the 3 hours, add the shredded cabbage to the water and simmer for an additional 30 minutes. Remove the corned beef from the water and allow it to cool until it can be handled. Trim off any visible fat and gristle. You should have about 1 pound of cooked corned beef. Drain the cabbage and set aside.

Puree the dill pickle in a food processor or blender. Cube half the corned beef and shred the other half. In a large bowl, mix the corned beef, pickle, and cabbage. Add pepper to taste.

Warm the butter in an 8-inch nonstick frying pan. Add the corned beef mixture and press down with a spatula. Cook over medium high heat until crisp.

Divide hash among 4 plates; top each with a slice of tomato and a poached egg. Sprinkle with the grated cheese.

## *Louisville Oeufs!*　SERVES 8

1　pound bacon
1　cup heavy whipping cream
1　dozen eggs
olive oil

6　ounces cheddar cheese, grated
6　ounces Swiss cheese, grated
1½　cups sour cream

Preheat oven to 350°. Mince the bacon (this will be easier to do if it is partially frozen). Fry the minced bacon until crisp. Whip the cream until stiff peaks form. In a separate bowl, whisk the eggs until pale yellow and then whisk in the whipped cream.

Spray a 9- by 14-inch baking dish with olive oil*. Pour in one half of the egg/cream mixture. Layer the cheeses over the eggs; follow with a layer of the bacon. Using a tablespoon, place dollops of the sour cream over the bacon layer. Top with the remaining egg/cream mixture.

Bake until set, 45 minutes to 1 hour. Cool for 5 minutes before serving.

---

*I recommend you make your own by buying a spray bottle (found in most cooking stores for this purpose) and filling it with olive oil. That avoids the propellants and other potentially hazardous ingredients in a commercial spray.

## Spinach Pie   SERVES 6

*(Also good as a light luncheon or supper entrée)*

1 pound Italian sausage
1 10-ounce package frozen
    chopped spinach, thawed
1 15-ounce container ricotta cheese
1 8-ounce package cream cheese

4 ounces shredded mozzarella
2 eggs, beaten
½ teaspoon hot sauce
2 teaspoons Italian seasonings

Preheat oven to 400°. Cook and crumble the sausage. Drain the spinach and squeeze it dry. Combine all ingredients.

Butter a 10-inch pie plate and smooth mixture in plate. Bake for 40 minutes until set and light golden brown.

Cool for 5 minutes before cutting into wedges.

## Benedict for the New Millennium   SERVES 4

4 large eggs, poached
4 slices Canadian bacon

4 portobello mushroom caps
2 tablespoons butter or olive oil

*Hollandaise Sauce*
4 egg yolks
8 ounces butter (2 sticks)

2 tablespoons fresh lemon juice
dash hot sauce

Prepare the Hollandaise: Melt the 2 sticks of butter in a small saucepan. Add lemon juice and hot sauce.

Put the egg yolks in a blender. As the blender is whirling the yolks, pour in the lemon/butter mixture. Continue to blend until the desired consistency is reached.

Sauté the mushroom caps in the 2 tablespoons butter or olive oil until tender. Warm the Canadian bacon. Put one cap, cup side up, onto each of 4 serving plates. Top the cap with a slice of bacon, a poached egg, and finally, top with the Hollandaise.

*Variation:* Omit the Hollandaise sauce and top with 1 ounce of your favorite cheese.

## Which Came First?   SERVES 4

1 pound boneless, skinless chicken breasts
2 cups chicken broth
1 cup sliced mushrooms
½ cup whipping cream
1 tablespoon minced fresh tarragon
    or 1 teaspoon dried

salt and white pepper to taste
olive oil
4 eggs
2 teaspoons minced fresh
    tarragon (if unavailable,
    use parsley)

Preheat oven to 400°.

Cut the chicken breasts into ¼-inch-wide strips. Combine the chicken, chicken broth, mushrooms, and 1 tablespoon tarragon in a medium saucepan. Add salt and pepper to taste. Bring to a boil and then simmer until chicken is tender, about 4 minutes. Remove the chicken and mushrooms from the stock. Boil the stock until it is reduced to ⅓ cup. Add the cream to the reduced stock and boil, stirring, until thick. Fold the chicken and mushrooms into the cream mixture.

Spray 4 gratin dishes or ramekins with olive oil. Using a slotted spoon, divide the chicken and mushrooms among the dishes. With a tablespoon, make a well in the center of each mixture and break one egg into it. Spoon the reserved sauce over the egg and chicken mixture.

Carefully transfer the dishes to a baking dish large enough to hold all four dishes. Pour 2 cups of water into the bottom of the pan.

Bake for 12 minutes. Garnish with minced tarragon.

## Sunday on a Wednesday Eggs  SERVES 4

### (Prepare this dish the night before.)

| | |
|---|---|
| 8 eggs | 1 tablespoon olive oil |
| ½ teaspoon ground nutmeg | ½ cup sliced mushrooms |
| salt and pepper to taste | ¼ cup chopped scallions |
| 2 tablespoons butter | ¼ cup sour cream |
| 1 tablespoon minced parsley | 3 ounces grated Swiss cheese |
| ½ pound Canadian bacon, chopped | |

Whisk together the eggs, nutmeg, and salt and pepper to taste. Warm butter in a skillet and scramble eggs until softly set. Stir in minced parsley.

Coat an 8-inch pie plate with butter or olive oil spray. Spread the eggs in the plate.

Sauté the Canadian bacon briefly. Place in a bowl. Sauté the mushrooms and scallions in the olive oil for about 2 minutes. Mix the sour cream, scallions, mushrooms, and bacon. Spread mixture over the scrambled eggs. Top with the grated cheese.

Cover with plastic wrap and refrigerate overnight.

In the morning, bake at 300° for 30 minutes, until lightly browned.

## Poached Eggs on Greens  SERVES 2

| | |
|---|---|
| 4 eggs | ¼ cup butter, softened |
| 2 cups arugula, loosely packed | 2 tablespoons minced fresh tarragon |
| 1 head (5-inch diameter) Boston lettuce | 1 tablespoon lemon juice |
| 2 tablespoons olive oil | salt and white pepper |

Poach the eggs and set aside. Clean the arugula and Boston lettuce. Tear into bite-size pieces and toss with the olive oil.

Cream the butter and mix in the tarragon and lemon juice.

Divide the salad mixture between two plates. Top each salad with two warm poached eggs. Divide the butter mixture equally and garnish the tops of the poached eggs with the butter. Season with salt and pepper to taste.

## *Baked Eggs*   SERVES 2

| | |
|---|---|
| 1 teaspoon olive oil | salt and pepper to taste |
| 1 tablespoon minced green onion | 1 ounce grated Parmesan cheese |
| 2 teaspoons fresh herbs | 4 large eggs |

Preheat oven to 400°.

Put ½ teaspoon olive oil into each of two gratin dishes or ramekins. Divide the onion and herbs equally between the dishes. Break 2 eggs into each dish over the herbs and onions. Sprinkle equally with the Parmesan.

Bake for 8 to 10 minutes. Season with salt and pepper to taste.

## *Basic Omelet*   SERVES 1

| | |
|---|---|
| 2 large eggs | 1 tablespoon butter |
| 1 tablespoon water | |

Whisk the eggs with the water. Warm the butter in a nonstick omelet pan. Pour in the eggs. As the eggs just begin to set, lift the edge of the egg with a spatula to allow liquid egg to slide beneath the cooked egg. Continue to cook over a low heat until eggs are set but not too firm. Top with desired filling(s) (see page 238) and fold omelet in half.

## *Basic Egg Roll-Up*   SERVES 4

| | |
|---|---|
| 6 eggs | salt |
| 1½ ounces grated Parmesan | 1 tablespoon unsalted butter |

Preheat oven to 375°. Beat the eggs with a pinch of salt and the cheese. Grease a jelly roll pan with butter, cover the butter with parchment paper and butter the parchment paper (as an easy alternative, you can spray the parchment with olive oil).

Pour the egg mixture over the parchment and bake for 10 minutes. Remove the egg roll-up from the pan and spread with filling of choice (see page 238). Roll the egg sheet as you would a jelly roll. Slice and serve.

# Omelet and Roll-Up Fillings

Once you have mastered the basic omelet and egg roll-up, the variations are limited only by your sense of adventure. Just make sure that the ingredients you use stay within the guidelines of the section of the diet you are on. The quantities below are for a roll-up. You may want to slightly decrease all ingredients for a single omelet. If you are cooking more than one omelet, the amounts listed below will suffice.

## Mushroom, Ham, and Brie

¼ cup sliced mushrooms, sautéed in 1 tablespoon butter
¼ cup minced ham
1 ounce Brie, cubed

## Artichoke

½ ounce grated Parmesan, mixed with 2 tablespoons Dijon mustard and 2 tablespoons mayonnaise
¼ cup canned artichoke hearts, drained and chopped

## Shrimp

¼ cup minced cooked shrimp
1 ounce cream cheese thinned with 1 tablespoon heavy cream
1 teaspoon Herbes de Provence (You can prepare your own Herbes de Provence by combining equal amounts of dried thyme, basil, savory, fennel, and marjoram)

## Florentine

¼ cup minced ham
¼ cup spinach, squeezed dry
½ ounce grated Gruyère cheese

## Italian

¼ cup cooked Italian sausage, crumbled
½ ounce shredded provolone cheese
1 teaspoon oregano
1 tablespoon minced tomatoes

## Shrimp Surprise

¼ cup diced cooked shrimp
¼ cup sour cream mixed with ½ teaspoon curry powder
1 teaspoon minced scallions

## Traditional
2  asparagus spears, blanched
½ ounce grated Swiss cheese

## California
2  ounces avocado, sliced
2  slices bacon, cooked and crumbled
1  tablespoon lime juice to sprinkle over the top as a garnish

## Nordic
¼ cup fresh salmon, poached and flaked, or 1 ounce smoked salmon,
   sliced in strips
¼ cup sour cream mixed with ¼ teaspoon dill to top the omelet

## Cowboy
2  ounces leftover steak, cubed
2  tablespoons chopped onion, sautéed in 1 tablespoon butter

## New Wave
3  ounces goat cheese, crumbled
¼ cup chopped zucchini, sautéed in 1 tablespoon butter
1  teaspoon rosemary

## Southwestern
¼ cup chorizo sausage, cooked and crumbled
1  ounce pepper jack cheese, grated

## Greek
1  ounce feta cheese, crumbled
1  ounce ripe olives, diced (about 4 jumbo)
1  teaspoon oregano

## Asian
¼ cup Chinese broccoli, blanched and sautéed lightly in sesame oil
½ ounce bean sprouts
¼ teaspoon sesame seeds to sprinkle on top

## ⊠ LUNCHEON RECIPES ⊠

## SALADS

### *Feta and Beef*　SERVES 2

12 ounces cooked rare roast beef
　　or London broil
olive oil
2 cups chopped field greens
3 tablespoons red wine vinegar

2 tablespoons oregano
3 tablespoons olive oil
½ cup diced cucumber
4 ounces feta cheese, crumbled
salt and pepper to taste

Cut the beef into small, bite-sized chunks. Spray a small nonstick frying pan with olive oil. Over high heat, sauté the beef chunks until hot.

　　Arrange the greens on a plate. In a small bowl, whisk the vinegar, oregano, and olive oil together. Toss in the cucumber, feta, and the warm beef. Scoop the beef mixture over the greens. Add salt and pepper to taste.

### *Lemon-Tarragon Chicken Salad*　SERVES 2

2 cups chicken broth

1 pound boneless, skinless chicken breasts

*Dressing*
½ cup mayonnaise (Hellman's or
　　Duke's has less sugar)
2 tablespoons Dijon mustard
4 teaspoons lemon juice
2 teaspoons lemon peel

2 tablespoons minced fresh tarragon,
　　or 2 teaspoons dried
½ cup diced celery
2 radicchio leaves

Bring the chicken broth to a simmer in a large saucepan. Add the chicken breasts and simmer until cooked through and no longer pink, about 7 to 10 minutes. Remove from the broth and cool. Once cool, shred the chicken. Reserve ½ cup of the broth and discard the remaining broth.

　　In a small, nonreactive bowl, whisk together the dressing ingredients. To thin the dressing, add chicken broth two tablespoons at a time, until the desired consistency is reached.

　　Mix together the shredded chicken, celery, and dressing. Mound on radicchio leaf to serve.

### *Babe's Cod Salad*　SERVES 2

½ pound fresh cod filets
4 tablespoons olive oil
4 tablespoons lemon juice

⅛ cup finely chopped parsley
salt and freshly ground black pepper

Bring a large frying pan full of salted water to a simmer. Slip in the cod filets and gently poach until opaque (do not overcook). Do not allow the water to boil.

With a slotted spoon or spatula, remove the filets from the pan and allow to cool. With your fingers, shred the cod, feeling for any stray bones.

In a small, nonreactive bowl, whisk the olive oil and the lemon juice. Stir in the parsley and then mix in the shredded cod. Season to taste with salt and ground pepper. Refrigerate for at least one hour to allow the flavors to blend.

## Salad Nicoise   SERVES 2

*Dressing*

| | |
|---|---|
| ½ cup sour cream | 1 teaspoon dill |
| ¼ cup chicken broth | salt and freshly ground pepper to taste |

| | |
|---|---|
| 6 ounce water-packed white tuna, drained | ½ cup fresh green beans |
| ¼ cup minced red onion | 2 hard-boiled eggs |
| ½ cup diced celery | 2 large lettuce leaves |
| | 4 jumbo black olives |

In a small nonreactive bowl, whisk the dressing ingredients until smooth. Flake the tuna and add to dressing. Add the red onion and celery and mix gently. Do not bruise the tuna.

Bring a small saucepan of water to a rapid boil. Plunge in green beans and boil for 3 minutes. Drain and cover with ice to stop the cooking process and to chill. Peel and quarter the hard-boiled eggs.

Put one lettuce leaf on each of two plates. Divide the tuna mixture equally and place on the leaves. Top each with 1 hard-boiled egg, half of the green beans, and two ripe olives.

## Cold Sesame Chicken Salad   SERVES 2

| | |
|---|---|
| 2 boneless, skinless chicken breasts | 2 tablespoons rice wine vinegar |
| ¼ cup minced scallions; use both green and white parts | ¼ cup lite soy sauce |
| 2 tablespoons creamy peanut butter, unsweetened | 2 tablespoons reserved chicken broth |
| | 1 cup broccoli, steamed and chilled |
| | 1 teaspoon toasted sesame seeds |

In a large saucepan, poach the chicken breasts in 2 cups salted water until opaque and cooked through, about 7 to 10 minutes.

Remove the breasts from the poaching liquid and reserve 2 tablespoons of the broth for the dressing. When the breasts are cool, shred the meat.

Put the next 5 ingredients (scallions through reserved chicken broth) into a blender and whirl until smooth (chunks of the scallion should remain). Toss the dressing with the shredded chicken.

Mound ½ cup of the chilled broccoli on each of two plates. Make a well in the center and fill each with half of the chicken salad.

## *Pretty in Pink*   SERVES 2

¾ pound shrimp, peeled, deveined, and cooked

½ cup red radishes, cleaned and trimmed

1 clove garlic

½ medium red bell pepper

⅓ cup mayonnaise

2 tablespoons raspberry vinegar

2 radicchio leaves

Chop the cooked shrimp into large chunks.

Put the radishes, garlic, and pepper into the bowl of a food processor or blender. Process until finely diced, but do not purée.

In a small bowl, mix the mayonnaise and the vinegar. Stir in the vegetable mixture and then toss in the shrimp.

Put one radicchio leaf on each of two plates, divide the shrimp salad equally, and place on each leaf.

## *Minted Lamb Salad*   SERVES 2

¾ pound cooked lamb

¼ cup fresh mint leaves, minced

3 cloves garlic, minced

¼ cup olive oil

2 tablespoons white wine vinegar

salt and pepper

½ cup cooked kasha

Cube the lamb and place in the container of a food processor. Dice, do not purée.

Whisk together the mint, garlic, olive oil, and vinegar in a small bowl.

Add salt and pepper to taste.

Toss the lamb with the kasha and pour the dressing over the lamb mixture. Toss again and serve.

# BURGERS

Any of these burgers may be made with any meat you desire. The recipes that follow give a variety of different meats. Feel free to change the meat in any way you see fit. All burger recipes make 1 serving, but may be doubled for two.

## *Louisiana Burgers*

¼ pound hot pork sausage

⅓ pound ground pork

2 teaspoons water

½ teaspoon hot sauce

Remove the sausage from the casing. Mix all ingredients in a bowl. Shape into a patty. Grill until cooked through, about 7 minutes per side.

## Burger a la Caesar

⅓ pound lean ground beef

3 tablespoons grated fresh Parmesan cheese

3 tablespoons mayonnaise

2 teaspoons olive oil

½ small clove garlic, finely minced

1 anchovy filet (optional)

freshly ground black pepper

1 cup mixed salad greens

Form the ground beef into a patty. Grill until medium rare, about 5 minutes per side.

Mix the next 6 ingredients (cheese through pepper) in a small bowl. Arrange the salad greens on a plate, top with the burger, and drizzle the dressing over the burger and salad.

## Top-Hat Burger

⅓ pound filet mignon, chopped finely, not ground

3 teaspoons finely chopped parsley

½ teaspoon Dijon mustard

2 egg yolks

½ teaspoon finely chopped shallots

½ teaspoon chopped capers

1 teaspoon salt

½ teaspoon anchovy paste (optional)

Dijon Cream Sauce (recipe follows)

Mix all ingredients in a small mixing bowl. Form the mixture into a patty. Preheat a nonstick frying pan on medium high heat. Add the patty and cook until it is medium rare, about 4 to 5 minutes per side. Remove the patty to the serving plate and top with Dijon Cream Sauce.

### Dijon Cream Sauce

¼ cup mayonnaise

1 teaspoon Worcestershire sauce

1 teaspoon lemon juice

1 teaspoon cream

1 tablespoon Dijon mustard

salt and pepper to taste

Using a wire whisk, mix first 5 ingredients in a small bowl. Season with salt and pepper to taste. Refrigerate until ready to use.

## Feat a Magic

⅓ pound ground lamb

½ ounce feta cheese, crumbled

5 medium Greek-style ripe, salt-cured black olives

Mint Sauce (recipe follows)

In a small bowl, combine the lamb and feta cheese. Chop the olives and gently fold them into the lamb mixture. Form into a patty. Grill the patty until medium, about 9 minutes per side.

Remove to a serving plate and top with Mint Sauce.

### Mint Sauce

    2  tablespoons sour cream
    1  small garlic clove, minced
    1  tablespoon minced fresh mint leaves
    salt to taste

Mix all ingredients and refrigerate until ready to use.


## South-of-the-Border Burger

⅓ pound ground beef                    ¼ teaspoon red pepper sauce
2  tablespoons onion, minced           ¼ teaspoon Worcestershire sauce
¼ teaspoon chili powder                cayenne pepper to taste
¼ teaspoon garlic salt

*Toppings*
1  1-ounce cheddar cheese slice        1  teaspoon chopped green chili pepper

Mix the burger ingredients together in a small bowl. Shape the mixture into
a patty and grill, about 7 minutes per side for medium rare. Top with the
cheddar cheese in the last minute of cooking time. Remove to a serving
dish and top with the chopped green chili pepper.


## Bangkok Burger

⅓ pound ground beef or turkey          2  tablespoons finely chopped cilantro
1  teaspoon finely chopped lemon peel  ½ teaspoon Thai fish sauce
½ teaspoon finely chopped lime peel       (use tamari sauce if unavailable)
¼ teaspoon Asian-style chili oil       Cucumber Salsa (recipe follows)

Mix all ingredients well in a small bowl. Pack well into a patty. On a ridged
grill pan, cook the burger to desired doneness (about 6 minutes per side for
medium rare beef burgers, about 10 minutes per side for well-done turkey
burgers).
    Remove the burger to a serving plate and top with Cucumber Salsa.


### Cucumber Salsa

    2  tablespoons seeded and chopped cucumber
    1  teaspoon Thai fish sauce or tamari sauce
    1  teaspoon rice wine vinegar
    salt to taste

Mix all ingredients in a small bowl. Refrigerate until ready to use.

# Chicken Licken

⅓ pound ground chicken
2 tablespoons diced red onion
2 tablespoons diced red bell pepper
2 tablespoons chopped basil
2 tablespoons cream

1 ounce Gorgonzola cheese, crumbled
⅛ teaspoon salt
⅛ teaspoon pepper
Licken Relish (recipe follows)

Mix all ingredients in a small bowl. Form into a patty and cook on a ridged grill pan to desired doneness, about 6 minutes per side for medium. Remove to serving plate and top with Licken Relish.

## Licken Relish

2 tablespoons chopped seeded cucumber
1 tablespoon minced fresh parsley
1 tablespoon minced fresh basil
2 tablespoons minced red onion
1 teaspoon lemon juice
1 ounce Gorgonzola cheese, crumbled

Combine all ingredients and refrigerate until ready to serve.

# Vegas Strips   SERVES 1

6 ounces chicken breast,
  cut into strips
1 tablespoon olive oil

2 tablespoons hot pepper sauce,
  such as Tabasco
Roquefort Dipping Sauce (recipe follows)

Put the strips into a plastic bag with the hot pepper sauce and marinate overnight in the refrigerator.

Heat the oil in a nonstick skillet. Over high heat, fry the strips quickly and remove to a paper towel to drain. Serve hot with Roquefort Dipping Sauce.

## Roquefort Dipping Sauce

1 ounce Roquefort cheese
2 tablespoons mayonnaise
2 tablespoons sour cream
2 tablespoons vinegar
salt

In a mixing bowl, cream the cheese with the mayonnaise, sour cream, and vinegar. Add salt to taste.

# SIMPLE CHICKEN TOPS

The following recipes are all based on grilled chicken breasts. To prepare, salt and pepper the breasts. Place on a nonstick cookie sheet and place under a broiler for approximately 3 minutes per side, or until cooked through. Alternatively, you may place them on an outdoor grill and cook through. All Chicken Tops recipes serve 1, but may be doubled for two.

## Veneto

1   6-ounce grilled chicken
    breast
1   ounce shredded mozzarella

1   tablespoon roasted sweet red pepper
    (from a jar)
½   teaspoon Italian herbs

Sprinkle the herbs over the grilled chicken breast. Top with the red pepper and finally the mozzarella. Broil until the cheese bubbles and is lightly browned.

## Heart-Art

1   6-ounce grilled chicken breast
¼   cup mayonnaise
2   tablespoons Dijon mustard

¼   cup canned artichoke hearts, drained
1   ounce grated Parmesan cheese

Chop the artichokes. In a small bowl, mix the mayonnaise and the mustard. Fold in the chopped artichoke hearts. Spread the mixture over the grilled chicken breast. Sprinkle with Parmesan and broil until the cheese bubbles and is lightly browned.

## Classic Chicken Melt

1   6-ounce grilled chicken breast
    (or turkey cutlet)
4   asparagus spears

1   ounce Brie, sliced
1   tablespoon chopped fresh sage

In a small pan of salted boiling water, blanch the asparagus spears for 3 minutes. Remove the spears from the water.

Top the chicken breast with the asparagus spears, then with the sliced Brie. Sprinkle the sage over the Brie. Broil until the cheese begins to bubble.

## Taxco Topper

1   6-ounce grilled chicken breast
¼   cup chopped tomatillo
½   teaspoon chopped jalapeno pepper
1   tablespoon lime juice
salt to taste

1   teaspoon chopped scallion
¼   teaspoon hot sauce
2   tablespoons mayonnaise
1   teaspoon chili powder

Mix the tomatillo, jalapeno, and lime juice in a bowl to make the salsa. Add salt to taste.

In a separate small bowl, mix the scallion, hot sauce, mayonnaise, and chili powder.

Spread the mayonnaise mixture over the hot grilled chicken breast. Top with the salsa mixture.

## Taj Mahal

1  6-ounce grilled chicken breast, chilled
2  tablespoons mayonnaise
½  teaspoon lemon zest
1  teaspoon lemon juice
¼  teaspoon dried dill

1  tablespoon chopped fresh mint
1  tablespoon chopped fresh basil
1  tablespoon chopped fresh watercress
1  ounce feta cheese (or, if available, use paneer, an Indian cheese found in Indian markets)

Mix the mayonnaise, lemon zest and juice, and dill in a small bowl. Spread this mixture on the chicken breast. Sprinkle the chopped herbs over the chicken breast and top with the crumbled cheese.

## Saltimbocca

1  6-ounce grilled chicken breast
4  sage leaves

1  ounce prosciutto
1  ounce grated Romano cheese

Top the grilled chicken breast with the sage leaves. Lay the prosciutto over the sage and top it with the grated Romano cheese. Broil until the chicken is warmed and the Romano cheese is melted.

## RAP & ROLL STYLE

These wraps can be made ahead of time, so all you have to do for a quick lunch is grab one. They are also easy to pack, so you can take them with you, wherever you or your family goes. All these recipes serve 2.

## Cyndi

4  napa cabbage leaves
4  tablespoons mayonnaise
8  ounces chicken breast, shredded

4  ounces avocado, sliced into 8 pieces
4  bacon slices, cooked
1  cup bean sprouts

Spread each cabbage leaf with 1 tablespoon mayonnaise. Divide the remaining ingredients equally among the leaves and roll up each leaf, jelly roll style. Secure with toothpicks.

# Carly

½ clove garlic
2 anchovy filets, drained
¼ cup mint leaves
2 tablespoons olive oil

1 tablespoon lemon juice
12 ounces cooked shrimp
4 napa cabbage leaves

Place the first five ingredients (garlic through lemon juice) in a food processor or blender and mix until smooth.

Coarsely chop the shrimp. Combine the shrimp and the mint mixture and divide equally among the 4 napa cabbage leaves. Roll up jelly roll style and secure with toothpicks.

# Luciano

¼ cup sour cream
1 tablespoon horseradish

4 tablespoons minced red onion
1 dill pickle, cut into 4 spears
2 ounces roast beef, sliced ⅛ inch thick

Mix the sour cream and horseradish. Lay the beef slices flat on a cutting board and spread the cream mixture evenly over each. Lay the dill pickle and the red onion on the cream mixture. Roll up jelly roll style and secure with toothpicks.

# Prince

8 asparagus spears
4 1-ounce ham slices

2 tablespoons Dijon mustard
4 1-ounce Swiss cheese slices

Steam the asparagus spears until they are crisp-tender, approximately 4 minutes.

Lay the ham slices flat on a cutting board and spread with the Dijon mustard. Top each ham slice with a slice of Swiss cheese and two asparagus spears. Roll up jelly roll style and secure with toothpicks.

*Variation:* Lay the ham slices flat on a cookie sheet and spread with the Dijon mustard. Top each ham slice with Gruyère cheese. Roll up jelly roll style and secure with toothpicks. Bake at 350 degrees for 10 minutes or until the cheese is melted.

# Janis

4 napa cabbage leaves
8 ounces cooked pork loin, diced
1 cup bean sprouts

1 tablespoon sesame oil
2 tablespoons soy sauce

Divide the pork loin and sprouts evenly among the four cabbage leaves. Drizzle each with the sesame oil and soy sauce. Roll each leaf up jelly roll style and secure with toothpicks.

## The Temptation

2 ounces crumbled blue cheese
2 ounces cream cheese
2 tablespoons sour cream

1 cup arugula leaves, chopped
4 napa cabbage leaves
8 ounces cooked London broil slices

Mash the cheeses together and add the sour cream. Continue mixing until smooth. Place the cabbage leaves on a cutting board and spread each equally with the cheese mixture. Sprinkle ¼ cup of the arugula leaves on each cabbage leaf. Divide the London broil equally among the four leaves. Roll up each leaf jelly roll style and secure with toothpicks.

## Diana

4 napa cabbage leaves
2 tablespoons Dijon mustard
1 cup watercress leaves

4 1-ounce slices Havarti cheese
8 1-ounce slices cooked turkey breast

Spread each cabbage leaf with ½ tablespoon mustard. Sprinkle ¼ cup watercress leaves over each. Top each with one slice of Havarti cheese and 4 slices of turkey breast. Roll up jelly roll style and secure with toothpicks.

## ⊠ APPETIZERS AND SOUPS ⊠

### Zucchini Spears  SERVES 4

2 large zucchini
4 ounces prosciutto

1 ounce grated Parmesan cheese
ground pepper

Preheat oven to 400°. Cut each zucchini lengthwise into 4 spears and remove end pieces. Steam over water for 3 minutes. Remove from the pan and allow to cool.

Wrap the prosciutto around each spear. Arrange the zucchini on a nonstick cookie sheet and sprinkle them with the Parmesan and ground pepper.

Bake for 15 minutes.

### Cheese Balls  SERVES 4

3 ounces feta cheese at room
  temperature
4 ounces goat cheese at room
  temperature
¼ teaspoon ground red pepper

¼ teaspoon ground cumin
2 tablespoons finely chopped mint
  leaves (or a savory herb such as
  thyme, oregano, or marjoram)
2 tablespoons olive oil

In a large mixing bowl, combine the cheeses with the pepper and cumin. Using a tablespoon, form the mixture into walnut-size balls. Roll the balls in the mint leaves. Refrigerate until firm. Divide the balls into portions and drizzle with olive oil.

## Spinach and Ricotta Dumplings   SERVES 4

| | |
|---|---|
| 8 ounces ricotta cheese | 4 jumbo egg yolks, beaten |
| 3 10-ounce packages frozen chopped spinach | ¾ teaspoon grated lemon zest |
| | 1 tablespoon soy flour |
| 3 ounces freshly grated Parmesan cheese | ⅛ teaspoon ground red pepper |
| | 2 ounces butter, melted |

Place the ricotta in a cheesecloth-lined strainer and allow it to drain for one hour.

Boil the spinach for three minutes in rapidly boiling salted water. Drain and squeeze until very dry.

Mix 2 ounces of the Parmesan with the drained ricotta. Add the beaten egg yolks, lemon zest, soy flour, spinach, and pepper. Mix well.

With wet hands (to prevent sticking), form walnut-size balls. Gently slip the dumplings into a large pot of boiling salted water. When the dumplings rise (2 to 3 minutes), remove with a slotted spoon.

Spoon the melted butter over the dumplings and sprinkle with the remaining Parmesan.

## Stuffed Mushrooms   SERVES 4

| | |
|---|---|
| ½ cup butter | 1 pound country-seasoned pork sausage |
| 1 teaspoon garlic powder | ½ cup minced parsley |
| 12 jumbo mushrooms | 1 ounce pepper jack cheese, grated |

Melt butter in a small saucepan and add garlic powder.

In the meantime, remove stems from the mushrooms and chop the stems into a fine dice. Remove sausage from casing. Cook the sausage in a large sauté pan, breaking it up as it cooks. Add the mushroom stems. Mix in the parsley and sauté until mixture is thoroughly cooked.

Swirl the mushroom caps in the garlic butter. Remove and place them on a nonstick cookie sheet. Mound the sausage mixture into the caps. Top with the grated cheese.

Broil until the cheese bubbles.

## Oriental Shrimp   SERVES 4

| | |
|---|---|
| 12 jumbo shrimp | ¼ cup rice vinegar |
| 2 teaspoons chili oil | 1 scallion, minced |

Clean and devein the shrimp. Using a sharp knife, cut partially through the back of each shrimp to butterfly them.

Warm 1 teaspoon oil in a skillet. Gently sauté the shrimp until they are opaque. Do not brown and do not overcook. Remove from the heat immediately and chill.

To make a dipping sauce, mix the remaining chili oil with the vinegar. Mix in the scallion. Serve the cold shrimp with the dipping sauce.

## *Bacon-Wrapped Scallops*   SERVES 4

| | |
|---|---|
| 12 slices bacon | 1½ teaspoons minced fresh ginger |
| 12 sea scallops | 1 scallion, minced |
| 2 tablespoons lemon juice | |

Fry the bacon until it is partially cooked. Cool.

Wrap one slice of bacon around each scallop and secure with toothpicks. Place the scallops on a baking sheet and sprinkle with the lemon juice and ginger. Broil the scallops, turning once, until they are cooked through, about 2 minutes per side.

Remove to serving dishes and garnish with the minced scallion.

## *Rosemary-Scented Zucchini Soup*   SERVES 8

| | |
|---|---|
| 2 tablespoons butter | 2 tablespoons chopped fresh rosemary |
| ¾ cup chopped onion | 3 cups coarsely chopped zucchini |
| 2 cloves garlic | ½ cup zucchini, cut in ¼-inch |
| 6 cups chicken broth | square dice |

In a soup pot, sauté the onion and garlic in the butter. Add the chicken broth, rosemary, and the chopped zucchini.

Simmer for 20 minutes until the zucchini is tender. Purée the soup in a blender. Return the soup to the pot and add the diced zucchini. Serve hot.

## *Cauliflower and Cheddar Soup*   SERVES 8

| | |
|---|---|
| 3 tablespoons butter | 3 cups chicken broth |
| ¾ cup chopped onion | 2 cups cauliflower |
| ¼ cup soy flour | 1 teaspoon Dijon mustard |
| 1 cup cream | 8 ounces cheddar cheese, grated |

Melt the butter in a large stock pot. Add onion and cook until golden. Stir in the soy flour and cook for 2 minutes.

Gradually stir in the cream and broth. Add cauliflower and bring to a boil. Reduce heat to low and simmer until cauliflower is tender. Stir in the mustard.

In batches, transfer soup to a blender and purée. Do not purée until smooth, but rather lightly to retain some texture. Return the soup to the pot and warm. Stir in the cheese until it is incorporated.

## Asparagus and Sesame Chicken Soup   SERVES 8

| | |
|---|---|
| 1   4-pound whole chicken | 3   cups chicken broth |
| 6   tablespoons sesame oil | 8   fresh asparagus spears |
| ¼   cup rice wine vinegar | 1   cup button mushrooms |
| 1   ounce fresh ginger, sliced | |

Discard the chicken neck and any organs that fill the cavity. Using a cleaver, hack the chicken into small pieces. Rinse with cold water.

Heat the oil in a wok until hot but not smoking. Add the chicken and brown. Transfer the chicken to a soup pot. Add the vinegar, chicken broth, and ginger. Bring the mixture to a boil and then simmer for 45 minutes.

While the broth is simmering, prepare the asparagus and mushrooms. Rinse the asparagus and cut it into bite-size pieces. Using a dry kitchen towel, clean the mushrooms of any dirt. Trim the stems. Quarter the mushrooms.

With a slotted spoon, remove the chicken pieces. Discard the skin and bones. Shred the meat and return it to the soup pot. Add the prepared mushrooms and asparagus and simmer an additional 15 minutes.

## White Gazpacho   SERVES 8

| | |
|---|---|
| 4   medium cucumbers, peeled, seeded, and chopped | 1   tablespoon white wine vinegar |
| 4   garlic cloves | 1½   pounds small shrimp |
| 4   cups sour cream | salt and white pepper |
| 5   cups chicken broth | ½   cup minced parsley |

Peel and devein the shrimp and remove the tails. Bring a pot of salted water to a boil and plunge in the shrimp. Boil until opaque, about 5 minutes. Drain and surround with ice to cool. Refrigerate.

Purée the cucumbers and garlic in a blender. In a large plastic bowl, combine the cucumber/garlic mixture with the chicken broth, sour cream, and vinegar. Add salt and white pepper to taste. Cover and chill thoroughly.

Before serving, mix in the shrimp. Garnish each serving with the parsley.

## Avocado Soup   SERVES 4

| | |
|---|---|
| 4   large ripe avocados | ¼   cup cream |
| 4   tablespoons lemon juice | ½   cup water |
| 2   small cloves garlic | cracked black pepper |
| 4   cups chicken broth | 3   slices bacon, crisped and crumbled |
| ¼   cup chopped onion | (optional) |

Pit the avocados and scoop out the flesh.

Put 2 avocados, 2 tablespoons lemon juice, 1 clove garlic, and 2 cups chicken broth in a blender. Whirl until smooth. Pour the mixture into a plastic refrigerator container. Repeat the process, adding the onions, and then whisk all together to combine.

Whisk in the cream and water. Cover and chill overnight. Add cracked black pepper to each serving.

Garnish with the bacon, if desired.

## Velvety Chicken Soup   SERVES 8

| | |
|---|---|
| 3 boneless, skinless chicken breasts | 2 tablespoons soy flour |
| 1 cup chopped onion | 6 cups chicken broth |
| 1 stick butter | 2 cups sour cream |

Poach the chicken breasts in simmering water for about 15 minutes. Remove from the water and cut into bite-size chunks.

In a stockpot, sauté the onion in the butter until the onions are soft. Add the flour and stir. Whisk in the stock. Transfer the mixture to a blender and process until smooth.

Return the mixture to the stockpot. Whisk in sour cream until it is incorporated. Add the cooked chicken. Warm the soup; do not allow it to boil.

# ▓ DINNER ENTREES ▓

## FISH

## Swordfish   SERVES 2

| | |
|---|---|
| 2 tablespoons lemon juice | 3 tablespoons olive oil |
| 2 garlic cloves, minced | 1 pound swordfish steak, 1 inch thick |
| 1 teaspoon dried oregano | ½ teaspoon olive oil |
| salt and freshly ground black pepper | |

In a small mixing bowl, combine the lemon juice, garlic, oregano, salt, and pepper. Using a whisk, beat in the 3 tablespoons of olive oil. Set the mixture aside.

Trim any darkened flesh away from the swordfish and discard. Heat a cast iron skillet until very hot and brush with the ½ teaspoon olive oil (or spray with olive oil cooking spray). Add the swordfish and cook over high heat until crusty brown on both sides. Remove to a platter and keep warm.

Add the lemon juice mixture to the pan. Heat quickly and thoroughly. Pour the sauce over the swordfish. Finish with a final grind of black pepper.

## *Sauteed Filet of Sole with Veggies*   SERVES 2

2  tablespoons butter
1  tablespoon shallots, minced
1  cup sliced mushrooms
1  cup zucchini, cut in a small dice

12 ounces sole filets
2  parsley sprigs
2  tablespoons diced tomato, as an
    optional garnish

Warm the butter in a medium-size nonstick frying pan and sauté the shallots over medium heat until fragrant, about 1 to 2 minutes.

Add the mushrooms and zucchini and sauté for 3 additional minutes. With a slotted spoon, remove the vegetables to a dish.

Add the sole filets to the pan and cook for 2 minutes. Gently turn the filets and spoon the vegetable mixture over the fish. Cover the pan and continue to cook until the fish is opaque, about 6 minutes. With a spatula, place the filets, topped with the vegetables, on serving dishes. Garnish each with a parsley sprig, and tomatoes, if desired.

## *Roasted Fish*   SERVES 2

5  medium black olives, coarsely
    chopped
3  tablespoons minced Italian parsley
½  clove garlic, minced
olive oil cooking spray
12 ounces cod or red snapper filets

⅛  teaspoon cayenne pepper
2  tablespoons olive oil
1  tablespoon lemon juice
1  teaspoon grated lemon rind
salt

Preheat oven to 375°. Combine the olives, parsley, and garlic in a small mixing bowl. Salt the mixture to taste.

Spray an ovenproof casserole with olive oil cooking spray. Arrange the filets in the dish and season with the cayenne pepper. Sprinkle the olive and parsley mixture over the fish. Pour the olive oil and lemon juice over the fish.

Cover and bake the fish for 30 minutes. Remove to serving dishes and sprinkle with the lemon rind.

## *Monk Kabobs*   SERVES 2

12 ounces monkfish (or other fatty fish,
    such as tuna or swordfish) filet
2  teaspoons Dijon mustard
1  teaspoon olive oil
1  tablespoon white wine vinegar
½  clove garlic, minced

¼  teaspoon dry mustard
¼  teaspoon cayenne pepper
¾  cup zucchini, cut into chunks
¾  cup mushroom caps
½  cup canned artichoke hearts, drained

Cut the fish into 2-inch cubes. In a large bowl, whisk together the mustard, olive oil, garlic, and vinegar. Add the fish and gently toss it to coat with the mustard mixture. Allow the fish to marinate for 15 minutes. Remove the fish from the marinade and reserve the marinade.

In a separate large bowl, mix the dried mustard and pepper. Add the vegetables and toss to coat.

Thread the fish and vegetables on kabob skewers.

Heat the broiler. Place the kabobs on a rack set over a cookie sheet. Broil about 3 inches from the heat. Turn after 6 minutes and baste with the reserved marinade. Continue to broil until fish is opaque, a total of about 12 minutes.

## Classic Salmon   SERVES 2

| | |
|---|---|
| 2  8-ounce salmon steaks | ¼ cup mayonnaise |
| 3  cups fish stock or fish bouillon | ¼ cup sour cream |
| (Knorr makes fish bouillon cubes that | 2  tablespoons fresh dill |
| are excellent for this usage; follow | ⅛ teaspoon white pepper |
| the instructions on the package) | |

In a sauté pan, bring the bouillon to a slow simmer. Add the salmon steaks and poach until cooked through, turning once. The total cooking time will be 15 to 20 minutes, depending on the thickness of the steaks. Remove the steaks from the poaching liquid and refrigerate until cold.

Mix the mayonnaise and sour cream until smooth. Fold in 1½ teaspoons of the dill and the pepper.

Remove the outer skin from the cooled steaks. Examine for any pin bones and remove them with tweezers. Decoratively slice the salmon and put on serving plates. Sprinkle the remaining dill over the sliced salmon and place a dollop of the dill cream on each plate.

## Oriental Shrimp and Broccoli Stir-Fry   SERVES 2

| | |
|---|---|
| 1  cup broccoli florets | 12 ounces raw shrimp, shelled |
| 1  tablespoon sesame oil (you may | and deveined |
| use chili oil if you like it spicy) | 2  tablespoons tamari sauce |
| ½ teaspoon grated fresh ginger | 2  tablespoons red minced pepper |
| ½ cup sliced scallion | (optional garnish) |

Bring a large pot of salted water to a rolling boil. Add the broccoli and blanch for 2 minutes. Drain and set aside.

Warm the sesame oil in a large, nonstick skillet. Add the ginger and scallion and sauté for one minute. Add the shrimp and stir-fry for 3 minutes. Add the broccoli and tamari sauce and stir-fry for 1 additional minute. Remove to serving plates and top with minced red pepper, if desired.

## ⬛ MEAT AND POULTRY ⬛

### Grilled Boneless Leg of Lamb    SERVES 8 TO 10

1   4- to 5-pound boneless leg of lamb, butterflied

Marinade
1  cup red wine                       5  cloves garlic
1  cup tamari sauce                   ⅓ cup fresh rosemary
½ cup olive oil                      2  teaspoons cracked black pepper

Place all marinade ingredients in a blender. Whirl until well combined.

Put the butterflied leg of lamb in a large self-closing plastic bag. Pour the marinade over the lamb and close the bag. Refrigerate the lamb overnight, turning occasionally. Alternatively, you may use a large plastic container.

Heat the grill. Discard the marinade. Place the lamb on the grill and cook 20 minutes. Turn the lamb over and grill an additional 20 minutes. Often the butterflied leg of lamb will be shaped irregularly, so cooking for 40 minutes will yield some meat that is rare and some that is medium well-done. That should serve your guests or family well.

Remove the lamb from the grill and allow it to rest for 10 minutes before carving.

### Lamb Chops with Mint Butter    SERVES 2

6  8-ounce loin lamb chops            salt and freshly ground pepper

Mint Butter
¼ cup fresh mint                     1  tablespoon coarse sea salt
¼ cup fresh parsley                  3  tablespoons butter

In a food processor or blender, chop the mint, parsley, and sea salt until the herbs are well chopped. Remove to a bowl, add the butter, and mix well.

Salt and pepper each side of the lamb chops. Grill them over high heat until cooked to your taste (about 3 minutes per side for rare). These may also be done in the broiler. Remove to serving plates and top with mint butter.

### Chicken and Sausage Bundles    SERVES 4

4  links Italian sausage             ¼ cup chopped parsley
4  6- to 8-ounce boneless,           ¼ cup fresh whole sage leaves
   skinless chicken breasts          ¼ cup dry white wine

Marinade
3  tablespoons olive oil             3  cloves garlic, minced
2  tablespoons lemon juice           salt and ground pepper to taste

Bring a medium-size pot of water to a rolling boil. Add the sausages and poach them until they are cooked through, about 15 minutes. Drain and cool.

Put all the marinade ingredients in a small bowl and whisk to mix.

Butterfly the chicken breasts, slicing as necessary to create a flat filet. Season with salt and pepper. Sprinkle with the chopped parsley and a layer of sage leaves. Position a sausage link across each filet and roll up jelly roll style. Secure with kitchen string. Pour the marinade over the chicken breasts and marinate for one hour.

Heat oven to 375°. Remove the rolls from the marinade and place in a covered casserole. Roast for 55 minutes. After cooking, remove the rolls to a cutting board and keep warm. Deglaze the casserole with the wine and the reserved marinade. Pour the mixture into a saucepan and boil for at least 5 minutes until desired consistency is reached.

Remove the string from the rolls and slice them on the diagonal. Pour the sauce over the slices to serve.

## Fourth of July Chicken   Serves 6

This marinade may be used for chicken, ribs, or other forms of meat that you and your family like to grill. For boneless country pork ribs, marinate the ribs for two to three nights and grill as you usually would.

Marinade

| | |
|---|---|
| 1 cup olive oil | 3 tablespoons sea salt |
| 1 egg | 1 tablespoon poultry seasoning |
| 2 cups apple cider vinegar | 1 teaspoon pepper |

6   10-ounce bone-in chicken breasts

Put all marinade ingredients in a blender and whirl until foamy white. Place the chicken breasts in a large self-closing plastic bag and pour the marinade over the breasts. Refrigerate overnight, turning the bag occasionally.

Heat the grill to medium. Grill the chicken until cooked through, about 15 minutes per side.

Remove from the grill.

## Chicken Sautéed with Raspberry Vinegar   Serves 4

| | |
|---|---|
| 2 tablespoons butter | ½ cup raspberry vinegar |
| 1 tablespoon olive oil | ½ cup chicken broth |
| 4 6- to 8-ounce boneless, skinless chicken breasts | ½ cup heavy cream |

Using a regular frying pan, sauté the chicken breasts in the butter and oil for 10 minutes. Remove the chicken from the pan.

Deglaze the pan with the raspberry vinegar and boil the vinegar down to 2 tablespoons. Add the chicken broth and return the breasts to the pan. Cover and simmer for 20 minutes. Again remove the chicken. Reduce the pan juices to about half.

Adjust the pan juices to taste, adding additional raspberry vinegar if needed. Add the heavy cream and heat until thick (about 3 minutes). Season with salt and pepper.

Slice the chicken breasts on the diagonal, arrange on serving plates, and pour the sauce over the meat.

## *Roman Turkey Cutlets*   SERVES 4

| | |
|---|---|
| 4  6-ounce turkey cutlets | 4  slices prosciutto |
| salt and freshly ground pepper | 1  tablespoon olive oil |
| ¼ teaspoon dried sage | ½ cup freshly grated Romano cheese |

Season the cutlets with salt and pepper. Sprinkle the sage over the cutlets and top each with a slice of prosciutto.

Heat the oil in a large, nonstick skillet. Place the cutlets in the skillet, turkey side down. Cook for 2 minutes. Top the prosciutto with the Romano and cover the skillet. Cook for an additional 2 minutes until the cheese has melted.

## *Horseradish Chicken*   SERVES 4

| | |
|---|---|
| 4  tablespoons white horseradish | 4  6- to 8-ounce bone-in skinless chicken |
| 4  tablespoons sour cream | breasts |
| 1  tablespoon Dijon mustard | salt and pepper |
| 1  tablespoon white vinegar | |

Preheat oven to 350°. In a small mixing bowl, combine the horseradish, sour cream, mustard, and vinegar.

Arrange the chicken breasts in a baking pan. Sprinkle with salt and pepper. Spread each breast with the horseradish mixture.

Bake for 45 minutes until the topping is brown and the chicken juices run clear.

## *Cornish Game Hens*   SERVES 4

| | |
|---|---|
| 4  Cornish game hens | 1  onion, quartered |
| 4  small lemons | olive oil cooking spray |
| 4  garlic cloves | salt and freshly ground pepper |

Preheat oven to 350°.

Rinse the hens and discard any innards in the cavities. Pat the hens dry.

Quarter each lemon and stuff each hen with 4 lemon quarters, one smashed clove of garlic and ¼ of the onion. Spray the hens with olive oil spray and then salt and pepper them.

Arrange the hens in a nonstick baking pan and roast for 1¼ hours, until the juices run clear. Discard the lemons, garlic, and onion. Serve hot.

## *Stuffed Chicken Breasts*  SERVES 4

*Stuffing*

| | |
|---|---|
| ¾ cup ricotta cheese | 1  10-ounce package frozen spinach, |
| ½ cup Parmesan cheese | defrosted and squeezed dry |
| 1  egg | |

| | |
|---|---|
| 6  6- to 8-ounce bone-in skinless chicken breasts | salt and pepper |
| | 1  cup dry white wine |
| olive oil cooking spray | |

Preheat oven to 350°.

Combine the ricotta, Parmesan, and egg in the bowl of a food processor. Whirl until smooth. Add the spinach and process until just combined.

Cut a pocket in each chicken breast and stuff each with equal amounts of the spinach mixture. Smooth the chicken down and secure the flap with a wooden toothpick. Add salt and pepper.

Place the chicken in a baking pan and pour the wine around it. Bake for 45 minutes. Turn the broiler on and brown the chicken for an additional 5 minutes.

## *Veal Piccate*  SERVES 4

| | |
|---|---|
| 1½ pounds veal scallopine | 4  tablespoons butter |
| 3  tablespoons soy flour | 1  cup dry white wine |
| ½  teaspoon salt | ½ cup chicken broth |
| freshly ground black pepper | 1  lemon, thinly sliced |

With a meat mallet, pound the scallopine until thin. Combine the soy flour with the salt and pepper in a plastic bag. Add the scallopine and toss until the meat is coated.

Heat the butter in a skillet large enough to hold the meat without crowding. Add the veal and sauté until brown. Remove the meat to a platter. Deglaze the pan with the white wine. Allow the wine to reduce, then add chicken broth. Return the veal to the skillet and heat until the sauce is bubbly.

Garnish with lemon slices.

## V's Arrosto di Vitello    SERVES 6

| | |
|---|---|
| 1  3-pound boneless veal roast | 1  cup sliced mushrooms |
| salt and pepper | 1  tablespoon soy flour |
| 4  tablespoons butter | 1  tablespoon fresh rosemary, minced |
| ½ cup minced onions | ½ cup white wine |

Preheat oven to 350°.

Season the roast with salt and pepper. Melt the butter in a skillet and sear the roast on all sides. Remove the roast. Add the onions to the same skillet and cook, covered, over low heat without letting them brown. Add the mushrooms and cook for 3 minutes. Sprinkle the soy flour over the mixture, then add the rosemary and the wine.

Place the roast in a baking dish and pour the mushroom mixture over the veal. Roast for 1¼ hours.

## Grilled Veal Chops    SERVES 4

| | |
|---|---|
| 4  6-ounce veal chops, 1½-inch-thick | 2  tablespoons olive oil |
| 4  tablespoons minced fresh rosemary | sea salt and freshly ground pepper |

Lay the veal chops on a cutting board. Spread 2 tablespoons of the rosemary over the chops and pound it into the flesh of the chops with the nonflat side of a meat mallet. Turn the chops over and repeat the process. Brush both sides of the chops with olive oil and season with salt and pepper.

Heat the grill to moderately high. Grill the chops to desired doneness, about 4 minutes per side for medium. Alternatively, they may also be cooked in the broiler, or in a grill pan on top of the stove. I would not recommend you fry these as they become very dry.

## Jamaican Pork Chops    SERVES 4

| | |
|---|---|
| 3  6-ounce pork chops | ¼ teaspoon cinnamon |
| ¼ cup coarsely chopped scallions | ¼ teaspoon ground nutmeg |
| 2  tablespoons minced jalapeno peppers | ¼ teaspoon ground cloves |
| 1½ teaspoons crushed dried thyme leaves | ¼ teaspoon ground black pepper |

Preheat broiler.

Combine all ingredients except chops in a food processor or blender and process until the scallions are finely chopped.

Rub both sides of the pork chops with the spice mixture.

Place the chops on the broiler pan and broil, about 2 inches from the heat, for 6 minutes per side.

## Herbed Pork Scallops   Serves 4

¼  cup soy flour
salt and ground pepper
1½ pounds pork scallops
3  tablespoons olive oil
½  cup white wine
2  tablespoons lemon juice

1  teaspoon lemon rind
2  tablespoons minced fresh parsley
½  teaspoon basil
¼  teaspoon thyme
¼  teaspoon oregano

In a plastic bag, mix the flour, salt, and pepper. Add the pork scallops and toss until lightly coated.

Heat the oil in a large skillet. Add the pork and cook until browned on both sides. Remove the pork.

Deglaze the pan with the wine and cook until reduced by half. Add the lemon juice and rind and the herbs. Return the pork to the pan and continue cooking until heated through.

## Stuffed Pork Loin   Serves 8

1  3-pound boneless pork loin roast
½  pound Italian sausage
½  cup minced onion
2  hard-cooked eggs

½  pound ricotta cheese
1  10-ounce package frozen chopped
    spinach, defrosted and squeezed dry
Fresh rosemary sprigs

Preheat oven to 350°.

Using a sharp knife, slice along the center of the roast to open it as if it were a book. Do not cut all the way through. Working from the center, slice each half again, forming a flat sheet. Season with salt and pepper.

Remove the sausage from the casing and crumble it. In a large skillet, sauté the onion and sausage for three minutes. Remove the mixture to a large bowl. Peel the hard-cooked eggs and chop them coarsely. Add the eggs, ricotta, and spinach to the sausage mixture. Stir to combine. Spread the mixture over the flattened pork roast. Roll the roast jelly roll style and tie it with kitchen string. Garnish with the rosemary sprigs.

Put the rolled pork into a roasting pan and bake for 1¼ hours.

## Ham Steak   Serves 2

2  tablespoons olive oil
¼  cup minced onion
2  cups shredded green cabbage
¼  cup chicken broth

1  12-ounce ham steak
¼  cup sour cream
½  teaspoon caraway seeds

Heat the oil in a large nonstick frying pan or wok; sauté the onion and cabbage for 3 minutes. Add the chicken broth and lay the ham slice over the cabbage mixture. Cover tightly and simmer over low heat for 20 minutes.

Remove the ham steak to the serving dishes and keep warm. Raise the heat to moderately high and add the sour cream and caraway seeds to the cabbage mixture. Heat through and serve beside the steak.

## Herbed Strip Steaks   SERVES 2

3  tablespoons assorted fresh herbs
   (thyme, marjoram, basil, parsley)
2  tablespoons butter, softened

2  6-ounce strip steaks
salt and freshly ground pepper

Mince the herbs finely and mix with the butter.

Preheat the grill. Generously salt and pepper the steaks on both sides. Grill to desired doneness. This can also be done in the broiler. Remove to the serving plates and top with the herbed butter.

## Senoran Steaks   SERVES 2

*Marinade*

¼ cup lime juice
¼ cup dry red wine
¼ cup soy sauce
¼ cup olive oil

2  cloves chopped garlic
1  tablespoon Worcestershire sauce
1  teaspoon jalapeno pepper

2  6-ounce beefsteaks

Put all marinade ingredients into a blender and blend until combined.

Put the steaks in a self-closing plastic bag and pour the marinade over them. Close the bag and refrigerate overnight.

Remove the steaks from the bag and blot dry with a paper towel. Discard the marinade. Grill the steaks to desired doneness.

## Babe's Eggplant   SERVES 2

1  medium eggplant
¾  pound lean ground beef
2  small eggs
3  ounces grated Parmesan cheese

2  teaspoons garlic powder
¼ cup chopped parsley
salt and pepper to taste
olive oil cooking spray

Preheat oven to 350°.

Bring a large pot of salted water to a boil.

Cut the eggplant in half lengthwise. Scoop out the eggplant flesh, leaving a ¼-inch shell. Drop the eggplant boats into the boiling water and boil for 3 minutes. Drain in a colander.

Cube the eggplant that you removed from the shells; you will have about 2 cups. In a large nonstick frying pan, brown the ground beef. Add the cubed eggplant and cook until the eggplant is soft and almost translucent. In a small bowl, beat the eggs and add the Parmesan, garlic powder, parsley, salt, and pepper. Add this mixture to the beef and eggplant. Using a spatula, turn the mixture over several times to mix.

Spray a nonstick baking pan with olive oil spray. Arrange the boats, skin side down, in the pan. Fill the boats with the eggplant mixture. Cover with aluminum foil and bake for 1 hour. Remove the foil and bake an additional 15 minutes to brown.

## *Beefsteaks with Gorgonzola Sauce*    SERVES 2

| | |
|---|---|
| 1 tablespoon minced shallots | 3 tablespoons heavy cream |
| 1 tablespoon butter | 1 teaspoon minced parsley |
| 1 teaspoon soy flour | 2 6- to 8-ounce strip or ribeye steaks |
| ¼ cup dry white wine | salt and freshly ground pepper |
| 2 ounces Gorgonzola cheese, crumbled | olive oil |

In a saucepan over medium heat, sauté the shallots in the butter until lightly browned. Sprinkle the soy flour over the shallots and stir for a minute. Slowly mix in wine and cook until reduced by half. Add the gorgonzola and stir until the cheese melts. Add the heavy cream and simmer for an additional 2 minutes.

Season the steaks on both sides with salt and pepper. Spray a cast iron skillet with olive oil. Heat the skillet until almost smoking. Sear the steaks on each side for 5 minutes for medium rare. Remove steaks to serving plates and spoon the Gorgonzola sauce over them.

## *Korean Short Ribs*    SERVES 2

1½ pounds flanken-style beef short ribs, ½ inch thick

*Marinade*

| | |
|---|---|
| 1 teaspoon sesame seeds | 2 cloves garlic, minced |
| ¼ cup tamari sauce | 1 teaspoon garlic powder |
| ¼ cup water | ½ teaspoon freshly ground black pepper |
| 2 teaspoons sesame oil | ½ cup minced scallions |
| 2 teaspoons minced fresh ginger | |

Put all of the marinade ingredients into a blender and whirl to combine.

Put the ribs into a self-closing plastic bag, pour the marinade over the ribs, and close the bag. Refrigerate at least overnight and up to 2 days. The longer the ribs are allowed to marinate, the more flavorful they will be.

Heat the grill. Drain the ribs and discard the marinade. Grill about 1½ minutes per side. Serve hot.

## Beef Stroganoff    SERVES 6

| | |
|---|---|
| 2 pounds filet of beef | 2 tablespoons tomato paste |
| salt and pepper | 2 tablespoons sour cream |
| 4 tablespoons butter | ¼ cup grated onion |
| 1 tablespoon soy flour | 2 tablespoons minced parsley |
| 2 cups beef broth | |

Cut the beef into thin strips and generously sprinkle with salt and pepper. Allow the beef to rest in the refrigerator for one hour.

Melt 2 tablespoons of the butter in a small saucepan. Add the soy flour and stir until smooth. Slowly add the beef broth and stir with a whisk to prevent lumps. Boil for 2 minutes. Stirring constantly, add the tomato paste and sour cream. Simmer gently.

In a nonstick frying pan, sauté the onion in the remaining butter until translucent. Add the strips of beef and fry until brown. Add the broth mixture and cover the pan. Simmer gently for 30 minutes. Garnish with the minced parsley.

## ⬚ VEGETABLES ⬚

### Gen's Green Beans    SERVES 4

| | |
|---|---|
| 2 cups green beans, washed and trimmed | 2 strips bacon |
| | ¼ cup grated onion |

Place the green beans in a steamer basket over boiling water. Cover the saucepan and steam the beans for 7 minutes until crisp-tender. Drain.

Meanwhile, fry the bacon until crisp. Remove bacon from the pan and crumble. Pour off all but 1 teaspoon of the bacon fat, and then sauté the onion in the bacon drippings. Add the hot green beans and toss. Remove to a serving dish and sprinkle with the crumbled bacon.

### Lemony Asparagus    SERVES 4

| | |
|---|---|
| 1 tablespoon butter, at room temperature | 1 tablespoon minced parsley |
| ½ teaspoon lemon zest | 16 asparagus spears, trimmed of any tough ends |

Using a fork, cream the butter. Add the lemon zest and the parsley.

Bring a large skillet of salted water to a rolling boil. Add the asparagus spears and boil for 3 minutes, until crisp-tender. Immediately remove the spears from the pan with a slotted spoon or spatula. Place the asparagus on a serving dish and spread the parsley and lemon zest butter over them.

## Squash Medley  SERVES 4

1 tablespoon olive oil
2 cups zucchini, cut into ½-inch cubes
1 cup yellow (crookneck) squash,
  cut into ½-inch cubes
¼ cup minced scallions

2 tablespoons vegetable broth or water
2 tablespoons minced fresh herbs
  (your choice—oregano, basil or
  thyme all work well)
salt and pepper

Heat the oil in a nonstick frying pan over medium high heat. Add the zucchini, squash, and scallions and sauté for 2 minutes. Add the broth and the herbs and salt and pepper to taste. Continue to cook for another 2 minutes, until all the liquid has been absorbed by the vegetables.

## Cucumber Sauté  SERVES 2

2 medium cucumbers
2 tablespoons butter
¼ teaspoon ground cardamom

¼ teaspoon white pepper
¼ teaspoon salt

Peel the cucumbers and cut them lengthwise in half. Using a melon baller or a spoon, remove the seeds. Cut the cucumbers in ½-inch slices.

In a large nonstick skillet, melt the butter over medium heat. Add the cardamom and stir until the mixture is fragrant. Add the cucumbers, salt, and pepper. Sauté the mixture for only 2 or 3 minutes, until the cucumbers are just warm. Do not overcook.

## Baby Bok Choy  SERVES 2

1 pound baby bok choy
2 tablespoons olive oil

1 cup chicken broth

To clean the bok choy leaving the head whole, rinse in several changes of water. Hold the leaves away from the stem and run cold water through the bok choy to remove any dirt. Pat dry with paper towels.

Heat the oil in a large, nonstick frying pan. Sauté the bok choy for 10 minutes, turning frequently. Add the broth to the pan and cover. Simmer for 7 additional minutes. Remove to a colander with tongs and allow to drain. Serve hot.

## Dressed-Up Cauliflower  SERVES 4

1 cup cauliflower florets, uncooked
2 teaspoons capers
2 tablespoons olive oil

1 ounce freshly grated Parmesan cheese
1 tablespoon minced parsley

Place the cauliflower florets in a steamer basket over boiling water and steam for 12 minutes, until crisp-tender. Remove the cauliflower to a serving dish. Drizzle the olive oil over the cauliflower and then sprinkle the Parmesan and parsley over the vegetables.

Serve hot.

### Baked Okra   SERVES 4

| | |
|---|---|
| 1 tablespoon vegetable broth | 1 pound okra, trimmed and left whole |
| ½ teaspoon melted butter | 1½ teaspoons minced shallot |
| ⅛ teaspoon salt | ⅛ teaspoon dried dill |
| ⅛ teaspoon pepper | 1 teaspoon lemon juice |
| dash Tabasco sauce | olive oil |
| 1 clove garlic, minced | |

Preheat oven to 450°.

In a large mixing bowl, combine all ingredients except the lemon juice. Spray a 1-quart baking dish with olive oil. Pour the okra mixture into the dish and bake for 30 minutes. Just before serving, sprinkle the lemon juice over the baked okra.

### Tropical Cucumbers   SERVES 2

| | |
|---|---|
| 2 medium cucumbers | 2 teaspoons lime juice |
| 1 teaspoon salt | 1 clove garlic, minced |
| 1 small chili pepper, seeded and minced | |

Peel the cucumbers, slice them lengthwise, and remove the seeds with a melon baller or spoon. Place them in a large bowl and toss them with the salt. Let them rest for a half hour. Pour the cucumbers into a colander and allow them to drain well.

Transfer the cucumbers to a serving bowl and gently toss with the chili pepper, lime juice, and minced garlic. Allow the mixture to rest at room temperature for one hour before serving.

### Cauliflower Latkes (Pancakes)   SERVES 4

| | |
|---|---|
| 2 cups cauliflower | 1 teaspoon minced parsley |
| 1 egg | salt and pepper to taste |
| ¼ cup grated onion | 1 tablespoon olive oil |
| 3 tablespoons soy flour | 2 tablespoons sour cream |

Trim away the center core of the cauliflower. Break the head into florets and cook in boiling water for 12 to 15 minutes, until tender. Drain in a colander. Using a potato masher, mash the cauliflower until the desired consistency is reached. If you prefer latkes with texture, leave a few lumps. If you prefer a smoother pancake, mash well, but do not purée.

In a large bowl, combine the mashed cauliflower with the egg, flour, parsley, salt, and pepper. Mix well.

Heat a large nonstick skillet and add the olive oil. Using a ½-cup measuring cup, drop 4 equal portions of the mixture into the skillet, forming 4 pancakes. Cook the pancakes until crisp and brown, about 3 to 4 minutes per side.

Remove to a serving plate and garnish each with ½ tablespoon sour cream.

## Brussels Sprouts Italiano   SERVES 2

1  cup Brussels sprouts
2  tablespoons Italian dressing, page 269

Trim the Brussels sprouts, discarding any discolored leaves and the tough stems. Cut in half lengthwise. Place the sprouts in a steamer basket over boiling water. Cover the pan tightly and steam for 5 to 7 minutes until tender.

Remove the Brussels sprouts to a serving dish and toss with the Italian dressing.

## Lemon Flowers   SERVES 4

1  cup broccoli florets
1  cup cauliflower florets

2  tablespoons butter, melted
1  teaspoon grated lemon peel

Place the broccoli and cauliflower florets in a steamer basket over boiling water. Cover the pot and steam the vegetables for 5 minutes, until crisp-tender. Transfer to a serving dish and toss with the butter and lemon peel. Serve hot.

## Sesame Spinach   SERVES 2

4  cups fresh spinach, loosely packed
¾ teaspoon sesame oil
1  clove garlic, minced
1  teaspoon tamari sauce
½ teaspoon sesame seeds
pepper to taste

Wash spinach, but do not dry it. Remove any tough stems.

In a nonstick skillet or wok, heat the sesame oil and sauté the garlic. Add the spinach and stir over the heat until it wilts, about 1 minute. Turn off the heat, add the tamari sauce, and cover the pan. Allow it to rest for one minute. Remove to a serving dish, sprinkle the sesame seeds over the spinach, and finish with a turn of freshly ground pepper, if desired.

## *Springtime Spaghetti Squash*   SERVES 6

| | |
|---|---|
| 1  cup cooked spaghetti squash | 1  garlic clove, minced |
| 1  cup broccoli florets | 1  teaspoon basil |
| ½ cup zucchini, cut into ½-inch cubes | ½ cup sliced mushrooms |
| 1½ tablespoons red wine vinegar | 2  tablespoons minced scallions |
| 1½ tablespoons olive oil | 1  ounce freshly grated Parmesan cheese |
| 2  tablespoons parsley | |

To cook spaghetti squash: Preheat oven to 350°. Cut the squash lengthwise and scoop out and discard seeds. Place cut side down in a baking dish, add ½ inch of water and bake for 45 minutes. Cool. Using a fork, pull the tines through the squash to create "spaghetti."

Place broccoli and zucchini in a steamer basket over boiling water. Cover and steam for 1 minute.

In a blender, combine the vinegar, oil, parsley, garlic, and basil. Whirl.

In a large bowl, gently toss the spaghetti squash, steamed vegetables, mushrooms, and scallions. Pour the vinegar mixture over the vegetables. Sprinkle with the Parmesan. Serve at room temperature.

**Variation on Springtime Spaghetti Squash:**

The recipe above makes 4 side-dish portions. To serve 3 as a main course: Remove the casings from two Italian sausages. Cook the sausage in a skillet until brown and crumble it over the Springtime Spaghetti Squash. Serve warm.

## *Spinach with Pine Nuts*   SERVES 2

| | |
|---|---|
| 4  cups fresh spinach leaves | 1  tablespoon pine nuts |
| 1  tablespoon olive oil | (also known as pignoli) |
| 1  ounce freshly grated Parmesan cheese | salt and freshly ground pepper |

Wash the spinach and shake dry. In a large skillet, heat the olive oil. Add the spinach and stir-fry it until it is just wilted, about 2 minutes. Remove from the heat and add the Parmesan, pine nuts, and salt and pepper to taste. Serve hot.

## ✖ S A L A D   D R E S S I N G S ✖

All salad dressing recipes make approximately 1 cup of dressing. The serving size for each is 1 tablespoon.

### Simple French Vinaigrette

| | |
|---|---|
| 4 tablespoons white wine vinegar | salt and pepper |
| 1 tablespoon Dijon mustard | ⅔ cup olive oil |

In a small bowl, whisk together the vinegar, mustard, and salt and pepper to taste. While whisking, add the olive oil in a stream.

Whisk until the dressing is emulsified.

### Gorgonzola Dressing

| | |
|---|---|
| ¼ cup red wine vinegar | ¾ cup olive oil |
| 1 shallot, chopped | 4 ounces Gorgonzola cheese |
| 3 garlic cloves, chopped | salt and pepper to taste |
| 2 tablespoons Dijon mustard | |

Place the vinegar, shallot, garlic, and mustard in the well of a food processor or blender and purée until smooth. With the motor running, add the olive oil in a stream. Put into serving bowl. Add crumbled Gorgonzola and stir. Check the seasonings and add salt and pepper as desired.

### Lemon and Dill Dressing

| | |
|---|---|
| 4 tablespoons fresh lemon juice | 4 teaspoons dill seed |
| 2 tablespoons white vinegar | 2 tablespoons mayonnaise |
| 1 teaspoon canola oil | ⅔ cup olive oil |
| 1 teaspoon dry mustard | salt and pepper to taste |

Put all ingredients, except olive oil and salt and pepper, in the container of a blender. Whirl until combined. With the motor running, add the olive oil in a stream until combined. Add salt and pepper to taste.

### Italian Dressing

| | |
|---|---|
| ⅔ cup olive oil | ½ teaspoon celery salt |
| ¼ cup vinegar | ¼ teaspoon white pepper |
| 2 ounces grated Parmesan cheese | 1 tablespoon Dijon mustard |
| 1 teaspoon salt | 1 clove garlic, minced |

Blend all ingredients in a blender or food processor. Serve chilled.

## *Lemon and Caper Dressing*

1½ ounces capers
2 teaspoons Dijon mustard
4 cloves garlic
4 tablespoons lemon juice
2 tablespoons chopped scallion, green part only (save the white part for another recipe)

1 tablespoon parsley
¼ teaspoon dried dill
¾ cup olive oil
salt and ground black pepper

Place all ingredients except oil in a food processor. Whirl until blended. With the motor running, pour in the olive oil. Blend until smooth. Adjust seasoning. (You may add more oil if the dressing is too tart for your taste.)

## *Fresh Herb Dressing*

½ cup olive oil
¼ cup red wine vinegar
1 ounce goat cheese, crumbled
1 garlic clove, minced
1 tablespoon Dijon mustard

2 tablespoons minced fresh thyme
1 tablespoon minced fresh marjoram
1 tablespoon minced fresh oregano
½ teaspoon white pepper
salt to taste

Place all ingredients in a blender or food processor. Whirl and serve.

## *Oriental Dressing*

5 tablespoons vegetable broth
3 tablespoons peanut butter, unsweetened
3 tablespoons red wine vinegar

6 tablespoons tamari
2 teaspoons sesame oil
3 scallions

Put all ingredients into a blender or food processor and whirl.

# ▧ GRAIN AND TOFU DISHES ▧

## *Kasha Salad*   SERVES 8

½ cup kasha, uncooked
½ cup grated zucchini
½ cup thinly sliced mushrooms

½ cup diced, peeled cucumber
½ cup minced scallion
¼ cup minced parsley

*Vinaigrette*
2 garlic cloves, minced
¼ cup olive oil

3 tablespoons red wine vinegar
salt and pepper to taste

Bring a pot of water to a boil and add the kasha. Cook until tender, about 15 minutes. Drain the kasha.

Put all the vinaigrette ingredients in a blender and whirl.

In a large bowl, mix the hot kasha with the vegetables and pour the vinaigrette over the mixture. The salad can be served warm or chilled.

## *Eastern Tofu*   SERVES 2

| | |
|---|---|
| 1 teaspoon sesame oil | 1 clove garlic, minced |
| ½ pound firm tofu | 2 tablespoons tamari |

Cut the tofu into 1-inch slices.

Heat the oil in a nonstick frying pan. Sauté the tofu for 2 minutes on each side. Add the garlic and the tamari to the pan. Cover and simmer for a final 2 minutes.

## *Southwestern Tofu*   SERVES 2

| | |
|---|---|
| ½ pound firm tofu | ¼ teaspoon red pepper |
| 1 clove garlic, minced | ¼ teaspoon black pepper |
| 1½ teaspoons paprika | 1 teaspoon butter |
| ½ teaspoon seasoned salt | |

Cut the tofu into 1-inch slices.

Mix all the spices together on a plate. Place one slice of tofu on the spice mixture and press until the spices adhere. Turn the tofu and repeat to coat the other side. In a large nonstick skillet, melt the butter and sauté the garlic until fragrant. Add the tofu slices and cook until golden brown, about 5 minutes per side.

## *Nutty Grain*   SERVES 10

This recipe can be used for most grains, such as brown rice, quinoa, amaranth, and so on, if you don't like millet.

| | |
|---|---|
| 1 cup millet | 3 tablespoons tamari |
| 3 tablespoons peanut butter, unsweetened (your choice, crunchy or smooth) | 1 tablespoon olive oil |
| | ½ cup minced onion |

Boil ¾ cup water and add the millet. Cook for 10 to 15 minutes until tender, not mushy.

Using a whisk, mix the peanut butter and the tamari.

In a nonstick skillet, sauté the onion in the olive oil until translucent. Add the cooked millet and toss to coat. Pour in the peanut butter and tamari sauce. Cook until hot.

## *Greek Quinoa*   SERVES 12

| | |
|---|---|
| 1 cup quinoa, uncooked | 1½ cups diced celery |
| 4 tablespoons lemon juice | 2 ounces goat cheese |
| 3 tablespoons olive oil | ½ cup minced parsley |
| salt and pepper to taste | ½ cup minced oregano |

Bring 2 quarts of water to a boil. Add the quinoa and simmer for 10 to 15 minutes until tender. Do not overcook. Drain in a colander. Cool.

Whisk together the lemon juice, olive oil, salt, and pepper. Set aside.

Mix the cooled quinoa with the celery, goat cheese, and herbs. Pour the lemon juice mixture over the quinoa and toss gently.

## *Minted Quinoa*   SERVES 12

| | |
|---|---|
| 2 cups chicken broth | 4 tablespoons minced fresh mint |
| 1 cup quinoa, uncooked | 2 ounces feta cheese |
| 2 scallions, minced | |

Bring the broth to a boil in a 2-quart saucepan. Stir in quinoa and simmer for 10 to 15 minutes until tender. Do not overcook. Drain. Fluff the quinoa with a fork and then add the remaining ingredients.

## *Fancied-Up Brown Rice*   SERVES 12

| | |
|---|---|
| 2 tablespoons butter | 1 teaspoon fresh chopped dill or |
| 2 shallots, chopped | ¼ teaspoon dried |
| 1 clove garlic, minced | 2 cups water or chicken broth |
| 2 tablespoons minced scallions | 2 ounces freshly grated |
| 1 cup brown rice, uncooked | Parmesan cheese |

In a large nonstick skillet over medium heat, sauté the shallots and garlic in the butter for 3 minutes. Add the scallions and the rice. Stir-fry the mixture until the rice threatens to explode (it will crackle, snap, and pop). Pour in the water and bring to a boil. Reduce the heat, cover the pan tightly, and simmer for 40 to 45 minutes. Do not peek. Remove from the heat, stir in the Parmesan, and serve.

## *Easy Pilaf*   SERVES 6

| | |
|---|---|
| 1 cup chicken broth | 1 tablespoon lemon juice |
| ½ cup brown rice, uncooked | 3 tablespoons sliced scallions |
| 1 teaspoon grated lemon peel | 1 tablespoon butter |

Preheat oven to 350°.

Mix all ingredients and pour into a 1-quart casserole. Cover tightly and bake for 50 minutes, until rice is tender.

## ❖ Desserts ❖

The sweeteners used in these recipes are liquid saccharin and stevia, the only noncaloric sweeteners available in the United States that I recommend. I think these sweeteners are the safest. If you wish to use other sweeteners, just use the equivalent amount—but no sugar!

### Creamy Strawberry Frozen Dessert   SERVES 6

2  cups diced strawberries                    ¾ cup heavy cream

Place strawberries in a food processor or blender and purée. Add the cream. Stir and pour into 4-ounce cups and place in the freezer. You can also place the mixture in an ice cream maker or in an ice-pop mold. Before serving, bring out frozen dessert to warm up on the counter for 5 minutes. This allows the creaminess to be more evident.

**Variations:**

Use puréed cantaloupe or watermelon, which kids really love.

- Creamy Cantaloupe Frozen Dessert: Use 2 cups ½-inch cantaloupe cubes in place of strawberries.

- Creamy Watermelon Frozen Dessert: Use 2 cups ½-inch watermelon cubes in place of strawberries.

### Mini Sour Cream Cheesecakes   SERVES 12

*For the crust*
4  tablespoons melted butter              20 drops liquid saccharin, or
½  cup miller's bran                            5 drops liquid stevia

*For the cake*
2  eggs, beaten well                          1  teaspoon lemon juice
¾  pound softened cream cheese           ½  teaspoon salt
1  tablespoon liquid saccharin,
    or 1 teaspoon liquid stevia

*For the topping*
¾  cup sour cream                            ¼ teaspoon vanilla extract
15  drops liquid saccharin,                 ⅛ teaspoon salt
    or 5 drops liquid stevia

First make the crust. Combine the melted butter with the miller's bran and add the sweetener. Line a muffin pan with paper baking cups. Put 1 teaspoon of the mixture in the bottom of each cup and press firmly to cover bottom. Refrigerate for at least 1 hour.

Preheat the oven to 425°. Combine all the cake ingredients and beat well with an electric mixer until smooth. Remove the muffin tin from the refrigerator and spoon the batter equally into the cups. Bake for 20 minutes. Remove from the oven and let come to room temperature.

When the mini cheesecakes have come to room temperature, combine the topping ingredients in a small bowl with an electric hand mixer until smooth and creamy. Glaze the tops of each cake with the sour cream mixture and place back in the oven for five minutes. Remove from the oven and let cool. Refrigerate for 6 to 12 hours before serving.

## *Snickersnoo*   Serves 12

This makes a lot of dessert. You may want to freeze half of the cauliflower or half this recipe if you are dieting by yourself, although everyone in the family will want to eat this—it is that good.

| | |
|---|---|
| 1  head of cauliflower | 1½ teaspoons cinnamon |
| 3  cups cream | ¾ to 1 teaspoon liquid saccharin or |
| 4  eggs | ½ to ¾ teaspoon stevia powder |
| 2  tablespoons vanilla extract | ground nutmeg, optional |

Trim the florets from the cauliflower. Place the florets into a food processor and run the processor in short on/off bursts until the cauliflower has a ricelike consistency. Boil in 2 cups of water for about 7 minutes. Pour out all the water and drain cauliflower well. Place the cauliflower back into the pot.

In a mixing bowl, combine the cream, eggs, and vanilla. Add this mixture to the cauliflower and cook for 15 minutes over low heat, stirring constantly. Remove from heat and stir in cinnamon and sweetener.

Cool before serving, and sprinkle the top with nutmeg, if desired.

## Nut Gems

*Serving size: 2 cookies. Makes 2 dozen cookies*

| | |
|---|---|
| 1  stick butter | 1  cup soy protein powder |
| 2  ounces cream cheese | ½ cup chopped undyed pistachios |
| 1  small package sugar-free | 1  egg |
|     pistachio pudding mix | 2  tablespoons unsweetened soy milk |
| ½ teaspoon vanilla extract | |

Preheat oven to 350°.

Soften butter and cream cheese and mix together well in a large mixing bowl. Add the powdered pudding mix and stir in until well incorporated. Stir in the vanilla, soy powder, and nuts.

Roll the mixture into 1½-inch balls and place ½ inch apart on a nonstick cookie sheet. Bake for 9 minutes.

## Strawberries with Almond Custard  SERVES 12

*Serving size: 2 tablespoons custard on 3 berries*

1 small package of sugar-free
  vanilla pudding mix
1 cup unsweetened soy milk

1 cup whipping cream
¾ teaspoon almond extract
2 pints large strawberries

In a large bowl, mix the pudding mix and the soy milk. Let this set for 5 minutes. Whip the cream in a separate bowl until it forms stiff peaks. Fold the whipped cream and the almond extract into the pudding mixture. Refrigerate for 2 hours. (This chilling is not absolutely necessary, but it will make the mixture that much stiffer.)

Remove the almond mixture from the refrigerator, take 2 tablespoons of this and place in a small serving dish. Fan a strawberry by slicing it several times but never all the way through to the stem on top of the custard and serve.

## Lemon Cheesecake Squares  SERVES 8

*Serving size: 1 1-inch square*

There can be many variations on this recipe, depending on what flavor you like. You may use different fruit-flavored sugar-free gelatins, but not puddings, for this recipe.

1 cup water
1 package sugar-free lemon gelatin

2 8-ounce packages cream cheese,
  softened

Bring the water to a boil in a small saucepan. Sprinkle the gelatin into the boiling water and stir until well dissolved. In the bowl of a standing mixer, mix the cream cheese until it is very creamy. With the mixer running, add the gelatin ¼ cup at a time. Mix until thoroughly combined. Pour into a 8- by 8-inch pan and refrigerate until firm.

## Peanut Butter Cookies

*Makes 2 dozen. Serving size: 2 cookies*

These are the simplest cookies you will ever make, and they sure do taste good.

½ cup unsweetened chunky
  peanut butter
¾ cup heavy cream
½ cup chopped pecans
2 teaspoons vanilla extract

½ teaspoon liquid saccharin or
  ¼ teaspoon powdered stevia
4 tablespoons soy flour
1 teaspoon baking powder
  (nonaluminum)

Preheat oven to 375°.

Place all the ingredients in a mixing bowl and blend well. Using 1 teaspoon at a time, roll the dough into walnut-size balls and flatten between the palms of your hand, and place on a nonstick cookie sheet. Bake for 12 minutes.

## Meringue's the Limit

*Makes 2 dozen. Serving size: 2 meringues*

| | |
|---|---|
| 4 egg whites, at room temperature | 10 drops liquid saccharin, or |
| 1 teaspoon vanilla extract | 2 drops liquid stevia |
| ⅛ teaspoon cream of tartar | 1 tablespoon unsweetened cocoa |

Preheat oven to 225°.

Mix the sweetener with the cocoa in a small bowl and set aside.

In a metal bowl, beat together with an electric mixer the egg whites, vanilla, and cream of tartar until it forms stiff peaks. Thoroughly combine the cocoa mixture with the egg whites.

Line a cookie sheet with wax paper. Drop the mixture by the tablespoon onto the wax paper and bake for 1 hour.

## Crepes du Jour   SERVES 2

| | |
|---|---|
| 1 large egg | ⅛ teaspoon vanilla extract |
| 1 tablespoon cream | Filling (recipes follow) |
| 1 teaspoon olive oil | |
| 10 drops liquid saccharin (this may be adjusted to taste), or 2 drops liquid stevia | |

Beat the egg in a medium-size mixing bowl. Mix in the remaining ingredients. Meanwhile, heat a nonstick frying pan on medium high heat. Pour half the mixture into the pan and swirl to coat the entire pan. Cook until this appears dry and then flip for a few seconds just to heat through. Repeat with the rest of the batter.

Place on a plate, add a filling (two are suggested below), and enjoy.

### Ricotta Filling:

⅓ cup ricotta cheese
20 drops liquid saccharin, or ⅛ teaspoon powdered stevia

Mix cheese and the sweetener in a small bowl. Add to the prepared crepe. This is enough filling for 2 crepes.

**Raspberry Filling:**
½ cup fresh raspberries

Wash the raspberries and place in a blender or food processor. Purée until smooth. This is enough filling for 4 crepes.

## Ace's Brownies

*Makes 8 brownies. Serving size: 1 brownie*

These are going to be somewhat different from brownies that you are used to. They are denser, not as light and airy, but they do the trick for a dieter who wants a chocolate fix.

⅔ cup soy protein powder
3 tablespoons unsweetened cocoa
1 teaspoon baking powder
¼ cup vegetable oil (I prefer to use olive oil, but if you think it may taste funny, try walnut or macadamia oil.)

3 large eggs
1 tablespoon unsweetened peanut butter
1½ teaspoons liquid saccharin, or 1 teaspoon powdered stevia
¼ cup water

Preheat oven to 325°.

Combine all the dry ingredients in a medium-size mixing bowl. Mix the oil and the eggs together in a separate bowl. Add the peanut butter to the dry ingredients and blend well. Add the oil/egg mixture and stir with a fork until blended. Add water a couple of tablespoons at a time and fold with a rubber spatula until the batter is smooth but thick. Pour into a nonstick 8- by 8-inch baking pan and bake for about 15 minutes. Allow to cool for 5 minutes, and then remove from the pan and place on a rack to completely cool. Cut into squares.

## Heidi's Sorbet  SERVES 8

*Serving size: ½ cup*

2 boxes of sugar-free gelatin, any flavor
1 cup heavy cream

2 cups boiling water
1 cup ice cubes

Place the gelatin in a large mixing bowl. Pour in the boiling water, stirring with a whisk. Add the ice cubes to the mixture and stir until dissolved. Add the cream and mix thoroughly. Pour the mixture into a covered plastic bowl and freeze until firm.

Remove the mixture from the freezer and place in the bowl of an electric mixer. Mix until the mixture is smooth again. Return the mixture to the plastic bowl and refreeze.

# Index